Clinical Governance

Clinical Governance

Improving the quality of healthcare for patients and service users

Second edition
Mary Gottwald and Gail E. Lansdown

 Open University Press

Open University Press
McGraw Hill
8th Floor, 338 Euston Road
London
England
NW1 3BH

email: enquiries@openup.co.uk
world wide web: www.openup.co.uk

First Edition published 2014, first published in the second edition 2022

A catalogue record of this book is available from the British Library

ISBN-13: 9780335251049
ISBN-10: 0335251048
eISBN: 9780335251056

Library of Congress Cataloging-in-Publication Data
CIP data applied for

Typeset by Transforma Pvt. Ltd., Chennai, India
Printed and bound by CPI Group (UK) Ltd, Croydon, CR0 4YY

Praise for this book

An excellent book for multi professional health care teams interested in quality in the context of clinical governance. Drawing on key theories related to quality in health care, the book provides an evidence based, step by step guide, to all components of clinical governance. It is a key text for both pre and post registration education programmes and also of interest to clinical staff involved in developing quality at all organisational levels, both nationally and internationally.

This second edition is written with reference to the UN's Sustainable Development Goals (SDG's) endorsing quality in health care; provides an updated evidence base; makes reference to pandemics, specifically COVID 19 and has developed discussion related to leadership.

Overall, a highly recommended key text for all those involved in quality in the health care arena.

Kathleen Malkin, Health and Professional Development, Faculty of Health and Life Science, Oxford Brookes University, UK

Praise for the previous edition

In this excellent new book on clinical governance, Mary Gottwald and Gail Lansdown distil down what this complex topic encompasses. They put bones on the individual components and lead the reader easily through the topic, so that he or she ends up with a good understanding of how the system is supposed to function and their individual responsibilities as a clinician, academic, trainer or manager ... I wish that I had been able to read a book such as this when I started off. It would have saved me a lot of time and trouble getting my head around all the aspects of this vital topic. Providing a reliable, safe, high quality service is the major challenge for all of us working in health services, so this fine book is very welcome.

Dr Peter Featherstone MPhil, FRCP, Lead for Clinical Governance in Acute Medicine

Consultant Physician and Honorary Medical Senior Lecturer Portsmouth Hospitals NHS Trust

The book has been developed for pre- and post-registration students, but it will appeal to a wider audience, particularly those who want more knowledge of governance and its antecedents. The outline of chapters at the start helpfully leads the reader to the appropriate section, and within each section the authors attempt to link clinical governance theory to practical examples. This is further emphasised by the use of reflective questions at the end of each chapter. The chapter on Clinical Audit is excellent and is of use to anyone including medical staff in terms of how clinical audit should be conducted.

It is an excellent, easy-read journey through all aspects of clinical governance and its application to patient experience, safety and effective senses, ultimately quality of care.

Sharon Linter, Director of Quality and Governance/Executive Nurse, Cornwall Partnership NHS Foundation Trust

Contents

Tables

Figures

Acknowledgements

The authors would like to thank the following individuals for their help during the writing of this book: Louise Collier and Debbie Hempstead for allowing us to use their SWOT analyses, Ed Gottwald for overall support, Patrick Henry for an introduction to values-based practice and how this supports evidence-based practice, Dr Marion Waite and Dr Louise Stait for their input on evidence-based practice, and Dr Helen Walthall for an insight into how education and training can be applied to practice. We would also like to thank Eldo Barkhuizen, our copy editor for the first edition and Dave Cummings, our copy editor for this current edition, for their invaluable help in checking our script prior to publication.

Every effort has been made to trace and acknowledge ownership of copyright and to clear permission for material reproduced in this book. The publishers will be pleased to make suitable arrangements to clear permission with any copyright holders whom it has not been possible to contact.

Overview of the book

This text, which will use working examples from practice, is primarily aimed at pre-registration and post-qualifying students studying on programmes such as Adult Nursing, Children's Nursing, Mental Health Nursing, Learning Disability Nursing, Paramedic, Midwifery, Operating Department Practitioners, Occupational Therapy and Physiotherapy. It will also be a useful text for staff new in post as well as staff moving into management, where an understanding of clinical governance is an important aspect of their role.

The idea for this text comes from our teaching experience both in the UK and Hong Kong at post-qualifying undergraduate and postgraduate levels. Our experience suggests that staff (i.e. post-qualifying students) are able to identify areas of practice where the quality of patient care could be improved. However, the assignments that we read consistently highlight that they find it difficult to take this one step further and are challenged in their learning and ability to apply clinical governance theories and strategies to their practice.

Since the first edition of the book was published in 2014, issues to be resolved within healthcare have escalated and the World Health Organization (WHO) has urged healthcare providers to be mindful of clinical governance. Added to this, health and social care organizations throughout the world have been faced with the further challenges of a pandemic. Furthermore, following a visit to the United Nations Headquarters in New York in 2019 and listening to a presentation on the Sustainable Development Goals (SDGs) outlined below, it has become even more apparent to us that the need to improve the quality of healthcare must continue to be a key focus for all those involved within health and social care.

Access to quality healthcare is a global issue but financial restrictions on the part of providers and/or service users can have a negative impact on the opportunities for such care. However, building on, developing, and strengthening existing healthcare organizations will help to ensure that practice is evidence-based. But without good leadership, this is unlikely happen. The World Bank and WHO have therefore made universal health coverage (UHC) a priority – in particular, services provided need to be of sufficient quality to have an impact on health improvements throughout the world. The WHO Global Monitoring Report (WHO and World Bank, 2017; 2019) identifies that millions of service users worldwide are faced with such high healthcare expenses that they can be forced into poverty. It also identifies that at least half the world's population do not have access to fundamental health services. The aim is to achieve UHC by 2030 (WHO and World Bank, 2017, 2019).

In 2015, the United Nations General Assembly identified 17 SDGs with the aim of improving health for all (the mantra of the Alma Ata Declaration of 1978). These goals are intended to help governments throughout the world to understand the need to improve the quality of healthcare provision. Targets to achieve these SDGs were identified. Target 3.8, identified as part of Goal 3 – Good Health and Wellbeing – is of specific importance to the application of clinical governance. The WHO and World Bank aim to support countries worldwide to improve their ability to implement governance strategies, thus improving the quality of healthcare provided. Progress since 2015 has been monitored, and the UN High Level Meeting on Universal Health Coverage held in September 2019 further endorsed the importance of political commitment to UHC. The International Universal Health Coverage Day is held annually in December, to act as a reminder of the need for access to health services for all and particularly those in the poorest populations (United Nations, 2020).

SDG Goal 3: Good Health and Wellbeing, Target 3.8

Target 3.8 of SDG 3 – achieving universal health coverage (UHC), including financial risk protection, access to quality essential health-care services and access to safe, effective, quality and affordable essential medicines and vaccines for all – is the key to attaining the entire goal as well as the health-related targets of other SDGs.

– WHO and World Bank, 2017: vii

Worldwide, healthcare providers are expected to meet this target and it is important to note that service provision is expected to be of high quality.

In total, 183 countries have contributed to the current UHC service baseline index which monitors Target 3.8 (WHO and World Bank, 2017). It is therefore important that all health and social care professionals reflect and consider what contribution they can make to achieving this goal.

The SARS-CoV-2 (COVID-19) virus has had a devastating global impact, leading to a pandemic unparalleled in living memory and globally has added further pressures on healthcare professionals to deliver and adhere to Goal 3: Good Health and Wellbeing. Not only has it put the greatest pressure on the UK NHS since its inception more than 70 years ago, it has also had a huge impact on healthcare organizations worldwide. Extensive changes to the provision of healthcare have enabled healthcare professionals to both cope with a marked escalation in demand for services, and to contain infection in the areas in which they work. Clinical governance, especially at a time of crisis, should support the improvement of the quality of services and safeguard high standards of care. To this end, the pandemic will be discussed in a number of chapters.

The rationale for this book

In the UK, there have been a number of high-profile cases in which the quality of patient care has been called into question. Cases involving Beverley

Allitt and Harold Shipman initially highlighted the need for well-defined clinical governance structures. Allitt, a State Enrolled Nurse, and Shipman, a doctor, were both serial killers who were convicted of murdering and attempting to murder children (in the case of Allitt) and adults (in the case of Shipman). It was because of cases such as these that the UK National Health Service (NHS) began to review its quality improvement processes to ensure that standards and quality patient care were achieved, and it was this that led to the implementation of clinical governance strategies. Whilst Allitt and Shipman triggered early thinking about clinical governance, further high-profile cases came to light. These included high mortality rates in A&E at Mid Staffordshire NHS Foundation Trust (2005–2009); Benjamin Green, the Banbury nurse jailed for 30 years in 2006 for killing two patients and attempting to kill 15 others; an outbreak of *Clostridium difficile* in Maidstone and Tunbridge Wells NHS Trust in 2007, in which more than 500 patients were infected leading to approximately 60 deaths where *C. difficile* was definitely or probably the cause; and Winterbourne View where a whistleblower reported that patients with learning difficulties were routinely being abused. The latter failure led to a government investigation and report and the hospital was closed in 2011. A mental health services review between 2014 and 2017 identified poor care and, more recently, the Shrewsbury and Telford NHS Trust (2017) was called into question regarding its care of babies and mothers.

Professor Liam Donaldson said that it is essential that practitioners learn from these errors because: "to err is human, to cover up is unforgivable, and to fail to learn is inexcusable" (cited in Fetherston, 2015: 27).

Following these early high-profile cases, clinical governance assumed as much importance as financial governance. We feel that clinical governance embraces three primary principles and these will be discussed in depth throughout the book:

1 High standards of care
2 Explicit responsibility and accountability for care
3 Constant improvement

We suggest that the following five components of clinical governance need to be stressed during a pandemic:

1 Health, Safety and Staff Management
   • Best underpinned through communication and policies designed to support staff wellbeing and a responsibility to slow the spread of the COVID-19 pandemic in 2020
   • Systems must be in place to contain COVID-19 and these must be freely accessible, thereby protecting the health and safety of healthcare professionals, their families, patients, and the general public

- The impact of sickness or quarantine needs to be mitigated as much as possible by clinical leaders, together with the possible necessary closure of other hospital clinical areas to facilitate an exponential increase in the number of COVID-19 patients
- Thought to be given to deploying the right staff to the right place
- Clinical leaders must be mindful of their responsibility to support accountability to protect staff and transparency to provide PPE to front-line staff in hospitals, care homes, and general practice surgeries. Nevertheless, there was a global shortage of PPE, with Cohen and van der Meulen Rodgers (2020) suggesting the following contributing factors in the United States:
  - Market and government failure to provide sufficient PPE during the crisis
  - Inadequate inventories of PPE due to poor hospital budgeting models
  - A failure of the federal government to maintain and distribute such inventories
  - Insufficient effort and policies to reduce dependence on the global PPE supply chain
    - (It could be argued that the same issues impacted on the supply of PPE in the UK and other countries around the world)

2 Risk and Crisis Management
- Government and clinical leaders need to take swift and decisive action
- Clinical leaders must ensure a crisis management plan is in place, and that it is robust. The pandemic was unpredictable and therefore attention needed to be focused on contingency plans, communication, accurate clinical documentation, bearing in mind data protection rules, and emergency succession plans should a key member of staff fall ill

3 Research
- The opportunity for research into pandemics generally and this one in particular

4 Audit
- Identifying lessons learned and ideas for continuous improvement to better manage the next pandemic

5 Clinical Governance and Ethics
- Healthcare organizations throughout the world are faced with everyday challenges to ensure that the quality of healthcare provision is constantly being reviewed and practice updated. However, during a pandemic there is a likelihood that there will be added challenges such as a tension between the ethics of good healthcare delivery and making humane decisions based on patient need and availability of resources

In consultation with many stakeholders, the Committee on Ethical Issues in Medicine of the Royal College of Physicians (RCP, 2020) issued guidance to frontline staff advocating that the principal values that inform any clinical decision should be:

Value	Description
Accountability	Ensuring ethical decision-making is constant throughout the pandemic
Inclusivity	Decisions are taken with appropriate stakeholders, whoever they might be
Transparency	Decisions should be publicly defensible
Reasonableness	Decisions should be made on evidence by credible and accountable staff members
Responsiveness	Decisions should be revised as new information about the pandemic emerges. Systems are in place to manage disputes and complaints

In respect of CQC regulatory requirements in the UK, it is important to ensure that arrangements are in place to meet regulatory compliance and assurance reporting. Equally, NHSE/I key standards need to be monitored and reported, streamlining reporting where possible and necessary.

With this in mind, the aims of this book are:

1   To provide readers with a text about clinical governance that is accessible and easy to read
2   To introduce students and practitioners to the practicalities of clinical governance
3   To enable practitioners to apply clinical governance theory and strategies to their practice
4   To show how best clinical governance practice can be applied to internationally common quality issues

Structure of the book

Each chapter follows the same format. Learning objectives are stated followed by a short introduction to explain the contents. In most chapters, key points and resources will be identified. In all chapters, activities will be included to guide reflection. At the end of each chapter, key points and implications for practice will be listed and finally some questions will be posed. The suggested answers to these questions are given in the Appendix.

Chapter 1

This chapter opens with a definition of clinical governance to help contextualize a number of issues that occurred between 1972 and 2021, and that had a negative impact on the quality of service provision in the UK National Health Service. The government's response to these high-profile cases together with their 10-year quality improvement programme using clinical governance is outlined. Clinical governance and quality are further defined and critiqued and our preferred definition of clinical governance is given. Finally, this chapter considers the engagement and involvement of service users/patients, carers, and the public in the provision and improvement of healthcare.

Chapter 2

This theoretical chapter sets the scene for quality issues that occur within practice both locally and internationally in acute community and mental health settings. It begins with an introduction to Never Events, Sentinel Events, and near misses. The chapter focuses on the incidence, morbidity, and mortality of eight quality issues that impact psychologically on patients/service users. The examples are taken from a variety of settings and include: needle stick and sharps injuries; hospital-acquired infections; ventilator-associated pneumonia; violence, bullying, and aggression; pressure ulcers; medication errors; falls in the elderly; and inpatient suicide.

Chapter 3

This chapter starts by briefly discussing clinical audit and how the audit cycle facilitates changes to practice. It goes on to explore how quality circles could be used to help health and social care teams initiate discussions around the quality of care provided. It explores and critiques a number of tools that could be used to analyse the reasons why particular quality issues and poor standards of healthcare arise in practice. These tools are applied to specific examples from practice. This edition includes some examples of a root cause analysis for medication errors and pressure ulcers.

The tools in question are:

- Maxwell 6
- Three organizational dimensions
- Ishikawa's fishbone
- SWOT
- PESTLE/PEST

Chapter 4

We have updated the title of this chapter so that an introduction to quality improvement programmes can be included. The chapter highlights some of the challenges and obstacles impacting on change and discusses how good leadership and management is needed as well as how change agents, advocacy groups, and the involvement of patients and service users can ensure the smooth transition of change. There are a plethora of change management models and this chapter considers five. Kotter's model has been included in this edition:

- The Diffusion of Innovation model
- Lewin's Force-Field Analysis
- The RAID model of change
- The Four A's model of change
- Kotter's 8-Step Process model

This gives practitioners a choice of models from the simple to the more complex. It is also suggested that a combination of models might help facilitate the management of change. The chapter concludes with an introduction to three examples of quality improvement programmes from the USA and UK.

Chapter 5

The focus of this chapter is on education and training – in our view, one of the key clinical governance strategies. Clinical governance and continuous quality improvement (CQI) can only be successful if healthcare organizations value their staff by putting structures in place. These structures are essential to empower clinical and non-clinical staff to engage in education and training.

Concepts of lifelong learning and continuing professional development (CPD) are explored, as well as the need for cultural change within health and social care organizations. VARK is discussed as a means to understanding one's own learning style, and practical suggestions on how education and training must be included at the individual, team, and organizational levels are considered. This edition includes a discussion on action learning sets. The chapter concludes with a look at learning organizations and organizational culture, and makes links to education and training.

Chapter 6

We have updated the title of this chapter to: "How clinical governance can be supported through evidence-based practice and values-based practice". The chapter focuses on the importance of both evidence-based practice (EBP) and values-based practice (VBP) and how these are applied to clinical governance. Also discussed is the link between EBP and integrated care pathways and care bundles.

Chapter 7

This chapter focuses on four approaches to quality:

1 Quality control (QC)
2 Total quality management (TQM)

3 Quality assurance (QA)
4 Continuous quality improvement (CQI)

Two further clinical governance strategies are considered, that is, risk management and complaints management. The similarities between risk management and quality assurance are discussed together with complaints management and shared governance.

Chapter 8

This chapter begins with a brief comparison of audit and research, which links to the discussion on evidence-based practice in Chapter 7. It focuses on how audit can be used to identify where there is a lack of quality care but also provide evidence on excellent care provision. However, it is important to recognize that EBP and audit have different functions. Three validated audit tools are presented together with a protocol for designing an audit. The audit cycle with prompts is discussed. Advantages, disadvantages, and barriers to audit are outlined. Finally, the chapter considers a variety of approaches that teams and individuals might consider.

References

Cohen, J. and van der Meulen Rodgers, Y. (2020) Contributing factors to personal protective equipment shortages during the COVID-19 pandemic, *Preventive Medicine*, 141: 106263. Available at: https://doi.org/10.1016/j.ypmed.2020.106263.

Fetherston, T. (2015) The importance of critical incident reporting – and how to do it, *Community Eye Health Journal*, 28 (90): 26–27.

Royal College of Physicians (RCP) (2020) *Ethical Dimensions of COVID-19 for Frontline Staff*. Available at: https://news.rcpsg.ac.uk/news/ethical-guidance-published-for-frontline-staff-dealing-with-covid-19-pandemic/ (accessed: 7 March 2021).

United Nations (2020) *International Universal Coverage Day 2020: Protect everyone*. Available at: https://www.un.org/en/observances/universal-health-coverage-day (accessed: 7 March 2021).

World Health Organization and World Bank (2017) *Tracking Universal Health Coverage: 2017 global monitoring report*. Available at: http://documents1.worldbank.org/curated/en/640121513095868125/pdf/122029-WP-REVISED-PUBLIC.pdf (accessed: 7 March 2021).

World Health Organization and World Bank (2019) *Global Monitoring Report on Financial Protection in Health 2019*. Available at: https://apps.who.int/iris/bitstream/handle/10665/331748/9789240003958-eng.pdf?ua=1 (accessed: 7 March 2021).

1 Clinical governance: the context

Mary Gottwald and Gail E. Lansdown

Chapter contents

- Learning objectives
- Introduction
- Working definition of clinical governance
- The birth of clinical governance
- Impact of poor care
- The government response
- Government White Papers and reports
- Defining clinical governance

- The framework of clinical governance
- Defining quality
- Linking quality and clinical governance
- Engagement of patients/service users
- Key points summary
- Implications for practice
- End-of-chapter questions
- References

Learning objectives

By the end of this chapter, the reader will be better able to:

- Understand the rationale for implementing a clinical governance framework
- Define concepts such as quality and clinical governance
- Critique definitions of quality and clinical governance
- Understand the importance of engaging and involving service users, carers, and the public in the development of health and social care provision

Introduction

A definition of clinical governance will be provided to contextualize eight issues that have had a negative impact on the quality of service provision in the UK National Health Service (NHS). These issues have been selected because specific reports have been published following government investigations. The government's response to these high-profile cases together with their ten-year quality improvement programme using clinical governance will be outlined. Clinical governance and quality will be further defined and critiqued and our preferred definition of clinical governance will be given. Finally, this chapter will consider the engagement and involvement of service users/patients, carers, and the public in the provision and improvement of healthcare.

Working definition of clinical governance

The first – and widely used – definition of clinical governance is that of the UK Department of Health (1998: 33):

> *A framework through which organisations are accountable for continuously improving the quality of services and safeguarding high standards of care by creating an environment in which clinical care will flourish.*

The birth of clinical governance

A number of high-profile and damaging incidents have occurred in the UK, some of which are outlined in Figure 1.1. Scandals such as these impact on the reputation of the NHS as a whole. We have selected adverse events for which inquiries and formal reports have been published, the latest being in 2020. However, there remain ongoing inquiries that we have not included. At the time of writing, Public Health England (PHE) is inquiring into deaths that occurred due to an outbreak of *Listeria* in 2019 in Liverpool and Manchester. Also, there is currently a 2021 inquiry, supported by the UK charity Birthrights (www.birthrghts.org.uk), into alleged systemic racism amongst the Black, Asian, and Minority Ethnic (BAME) community who do not receive the respect and dignity they deserve in pregnancy and childbirth. Research that will be included in this inquiry was initially carried out by Henderson, Gau, and Redshaw (2013). A secondary analysis using a questionnaire survey of 24,319 women, with a response rate of 52%, concluded that BAME women had a much more negative experience throughout their maternity care. There were statistically significant differences, with the BAME community less likely to be given pethidine and more likely to have a caesarean section than their white counterparts. They felt they were left alone during and just after giving birth, causing them worry and therefore a more negative experience. Overall, the results demonstrated that whilst women in all BAME groups experienced racism, there was a clear lack of recognition of diversity, cultural and religious beliefs between Asian and Black women as well as between women in all BAME groups compared with white women.

The Bristol Royal Infirmary

It was identified that over a 10-year period from 1984 to 1995, the care of children who required complex cardiac surgery was compromised and the mortality rate was approximately double the national average.

Dr Harold Shipman

Shipman was a respected general practitioner from Hyde in Greater Manchester who was thought to be responsible for murdering in the region of 215 patients between 1972 and 1998. Following a trial in 2000, he was charged with 15 counts of murder and was sentenced to life in prison. He committed suicide in prison in January 2004.

Nurse Beverley Allitt

Allitt was employed as a junior nurse on the paediatric ward at Grantham and Kesteven General Hospital and between February and April 1991 she injured eight children; she murdered four and was also found guilty of four counts of attempted murder of children whilst in her care. She was diagnosed with Munchhausen Syndrome by Proxy. Allitt is currently serving three life sentences.

Maidstone and Tunbridge Wells NHS Trust

Between 2004 and 2006, approximately 60 fatalities were identified where *Clostridium difficile* was definitely or probably the cause of death. A lack of infection prevention and control procedures was cited.

Mid Staffordshire NHS Foundation Trust

Between 2005 and 2009, there was a failure to provide high standards of care, which led to patients being put at risk and a high mortality rate. The campaigning group Cure the NHS helped to reveal that patients and relatives experienced poor quality care, such as patients being left in soiled bedding, not being helped at mealtimes, privacy and dignity not being respected, and a lack of compassion and candour on the part of staff.

Winterbourne View

Winterbourne View was a private hospital that provided assessment, treatment, and rehabilitation for individuals with learning disabilities. Although a whistleblower voiced concerns, these were not acted upon and it took a television documentary to uncover a culture of abuse, both physical and emotional. This led to the hospital's closure in 2011.

Mental Health Services (England)

Between 2014 and 2017, the Care Quality Commission (CQC, 2017) carried out a comprehensive inspection of all specialist mental health services in England. They evaluated various aspects that included:

* Safety of service
* Restrictions imposed on patients
* Access and waiting times
* Poor clinical information systems

Fifty-four NHS Trusts and 221 independent mental health services were inspected. The CQC reported that 36% of core NHS services and 34% of independent mental health services were rated as requiring improvement. In addition, 4% of NHS services and 5% of independent mental health services were rated as inadequate. Findings included locked rehabilitation wards, patients not being provided with relevant skills to empower them to live more independently, and some staff not having the skills required.

Shrewsbury and Telford Hospital NHS Trust

In 2017, families raised concerns with regards to the maternity unit where babies and mothers either died or experienced serious harm.

Impact of poor care

Although a number of significant events occurred in the UK that ultimately led to the implementation of clinical governance (Figure 1.1), staff commitment was not called into question in any of the above cases. As identified by the Francis Report (2013), the problem was generally a lack of leadership, ineffective communication, poor organization and teamwork, and a lack of means for assessing the quality of care.

One area where the impact of poor care is particularly evident is medical errors. Medical errors are linked to a high incidence of morbidity, mortality, and a financial burden throughout the world. According to the WHO (2019), globally the cost of medical errors is US$42 billion per annum. The UK Department of Health identified that "10% of inpatient adverse events resulted in harm to patients and approximately half of these errors were avoidable" (2000: 11). According to Slawomirski, Auraaen, and Klazinga, there are 134 million adverse events annually in low- and middle-income countries and "patient harm is estimated to be the 14th leading cause of the global disease burden" (2017: 6).

Figure 1.1 Examples of poor quality care

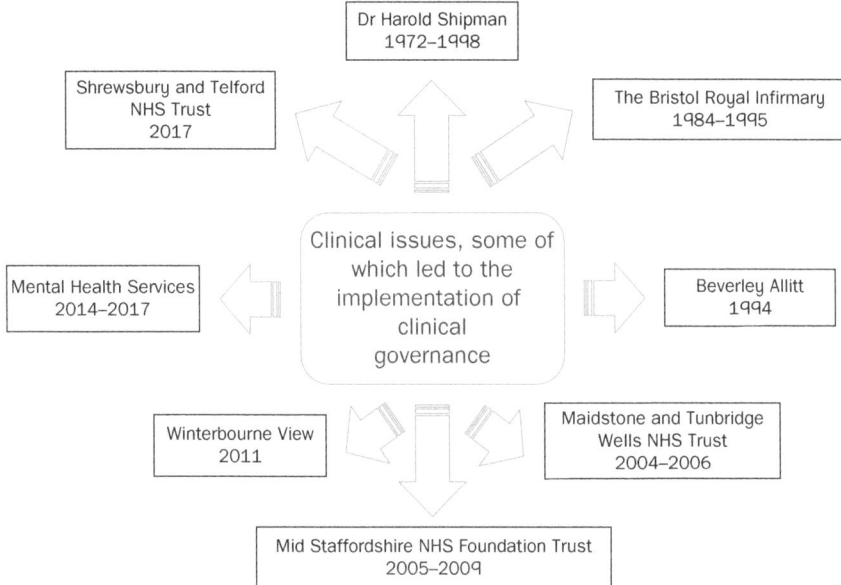

Adapted from: MacDonald (1996), Secretary of State for Health (2001), Department of Health (2006, 2012c), Healthcare Commission (2007), The Francis Report (2013), NHS (2014), The Ockendon Report (2020).

Also the WHO (2019) states there is a 1 in 300 chance that an error will occur and a patient will be harmed whilst receiving a health intervention. From the above, it is evident that adverse events are a serious issue.

Claims between 1998 and 1999 from adverse events cost the NHS approximately £400 million. However, between 2019 and 2020 that figure rose to £84.1 billion (NHS Resolution, 2020). Fetherston (2015) states that the WHO estimates that between 20% and 40% of healthcare costs worldwide are wasted because of poor quality care. The WHO (2017) goes further and states that poor quality care accounts for 10% of hospital deaths and patients left disabled. The WHO (2019) is proposing that, globally, medical errors should be reduced by 50%.

The effects of experiencing poor quality care, whatever they might be, and any possible litigation process will have an impact on service users'/patients' as well as staff's physical, emotional, and psychological wellbeing. This is clearly an ineffective use of public money and supports the continued need to implement quality improvement programmes through clinical governance.

The government response

The government responded to each of the high-profile cases outlined above (see Figure 1.2).

Figure 1.2 Government responses to these incidents

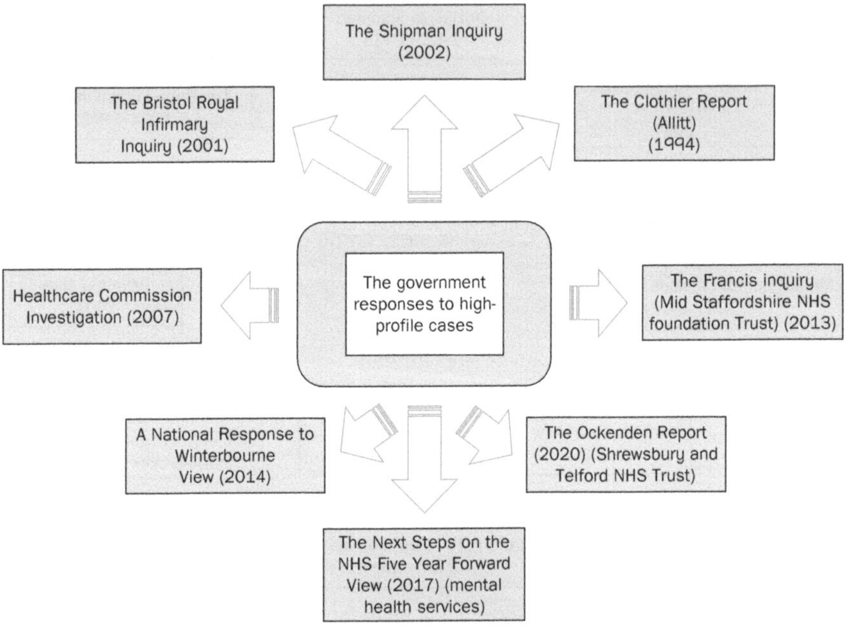

The Clothier Report (1994) on Beverley Allitt

Owing to Allitt's psychological disorder, the central responsibility lay with Allitt. However, the report identified failures of management and communications within the hospital. Both the School of Nursing and the Occupational Health Department within the hospital knew of her psychiatric disturbance and yet she was still employed to work in a paediatric unit.

The Bristol Royal Infirmary Inquiry (2001)

The public inquiry was the largest investigation into medical standards of care in the NHS at that time, and was conducted between 1991 and 2001 and divided into two phases. Phase 1 focused on the events in Bristol while Phase 2 focused on the future. The report contained nearly 200 recommendations including better identification of the needs of very sick children, the safety arrangements for caring for very sick children, the competence of healthcare professionals (and their terms of employment to ensure equity between consultants, nurses, and managers), standards of care, openness and monitoring of clinical performance, and improved leadership and teamwork.

The Shipman Inquiry (Smith, 2002)

The Shipman Inquiry was set up in January 2001 as a result of Shipman's conviction in 2000 for the murder of 15 of his patients. A total of six reports were published. The first and last reports examined Shipman's criminal activities as a general practitioner (GP). The other reports examined the processes and systems that failed to identify his activities (the second report looked at Greater Manchester Police, the third report the coroner's system, the fourth report the safe and appropriate use of controlled drugs, and the fifth report looked at monitoring and disciplining GPs, whistleblowing, and the handling of complaints in the NHS).

The Healthcare Commission's Report (2007) on Maidstone and Tonbridge Wells NHS Trust

The Healthcare Commission carried out an investigation between 2006 and 2007 into outbreaks of *Clostridium difficile*. The Trust had a relatively high rate of infection and this doubled in the autumn of 2005, although this was not acknowledged at the time. It was identified that the guidelines for management of patients with *C. difficile* did not highlight the importance of isolation of patients with infection. The infection control team were aware of this but there were not enough side rooms available and therefore patients with *C. difficile* were nursed on open wards. The Trust's policy on responding to outbreaks was not considered fit for purpose.

Transforming Care: A national response to Winterbourne View Hospital (Department of Health, 2012c)

The final Department of Health report was published following successful criminal proceedings against some members of staff. Findings of the report identified the poor quality of care provided at Winterbourne View, which included individuals being restrained unnecessarily, family members not being allowed to visit wards or bedrooms of their loved ones, and the poor management of complaints. The review considered how people with challenging behaviours could be better supported throughout England and included a review by the Care Quality Commission of 150 hospitals for persons with learning disabilities and autism who were admitted under the Mental Health Act. This report led to a programme for change and stated that individuals should have personalized care and either live at home or in the community near to their home and family. Additionally, and as a result, the Department of Health established Safeguarding Boards for Adults. Since 2013, Higher Education England has had a duty to ensure that providers involve people with learning disabilities and autism and their families in evaluating the quality of services provided. Providers are also expected to ensure that there is a sufficient workforce and that the staff employed have the right training, skills, and shared values (Department of Health, 2012c).

The Francis Report (2013) on Mid Staffordshire NHS Foundation Trust

This report identified a number of warning signs such as an organizational culture that did not focus on patients (organizational culture will be discussed in more depth in Chapter 5) and a culture that focused on positive information about the service rather than issues that were causing concern. The inquiry findings showed that staff were too tolerant of poor standards that put patients at risk, there was a failure to communicate by those who had concerns, monitoring performance management or intervention was seen as someone else's responsibility, and there was also the impact of repeated organizational changes. Once again, a number of recommendations were made, in this case 290 in total. The key recommendations included a single regulator for financial and care quality, more power to suspend or prosecute hospital boards and individuals, a duty of candour, gagging clauses to be banned in policies and contracts, only registered healthcare professionals ought to care for patients, clearer leadership to ensure clarity of who is in overall charge of patient care, complaints to be published on hospital websites, and GPs should monitor their patients receiving secondary care.

Mental Health Services (England) (2017)

The *Five Year Forward View* (NHS, 2014) was published to facilitate continued development of mental health services. *The Next Steps on the Five Year Forward View* (NHS, 2017) shows that changes within mental health services have led to better quality care. Some examples of changes include new mother and baby mental health units, the development of specialist perinatal mental health teams, improved care for children and young people, care to be provided nearer to home, and the establishment of 24-hour mental health teams (NHS, 2017).

The Ockenden Report (2020) on Shrewsbury and Telford Hospital NHS Trust

Published in 2020, this first report reviewed 250 cases and contacts with over 800 families. A second more in-depth and detailed report is due in 2021 and will include the review of just under 2,000 families. This independent review, chaired by Donna Ockenden, focused on all reported cases of maternal and neonatal harm between 2000 and 2019, including neonatal and maternal deaths as well as complications with adverse outcomes for both mothers and babies. The implementation of seven essential actions was deemed necessary (Ockenden Report, 2020: 26–30):

1 Enhanced safety
2 Listening to women and families
3 Staff training and working together
4 Managing complex pregnancy
5 Risk assessment throughout pregnancy
6 Monitoring foetal wellbeing
7 Informed consent

Government White Papers and reports

Not only did the government set up inquiries to deal with each of the critical incidents outlined above, they also published a number of government White Papers in which the recommendations were enshrined.

It was after the recognized high paediatric mortality rates in Bristol and the deaths caused by Beverley Allitt and Dr Harold Shipman that the UK Department of Health White Paper, *The New NHS: Modern, Dependable* (1997), began to address the need to improve the quality of healthcare. The following year, *A First Class Service: Quality in the New NHS* (Department of Health, 1998) outlined the then government's strategy for ensuring quality care was provided for all. The *Five Year Forward View* (NHS, 2014) set out the national plan to improve the quality of care and improve financial efficiency within services in England.

These papers identified a 10-year programme that would have quality at the centre of the UK National Health Service and would lead to guaranteed national standards of excellence. The aim of this quality service was to ensure that healthcare professionals would be "doing the right things, at the right time, for the right people, and doing them right – first time" (Department of Health 1997: Part 3). *The NHS Long Term Plan* (NHS, 2019) identifies how the NHS will move towards a new service model which will give service users more choice and improved support. It also includes plans to reduce health inequalities, improve the quality of care and patient outcomes. Staff experiences and well-being are equally important to the patient experience and this report discusses how the challenges of workforce pressures will be confronted (NHS, 2019).

It was after 1997 that a system of clinical governance in all NHS Trusts was introduced so as to guarantee patient safety and quality care, with "a formal responsibility for quality ... placed on every health organisation in the country through arrangements for clinical governance at local level" (Department of Health, 2000: 1). Briefly, clinical governance was an "organisational concept" (Department of Health, 2000: 2) that facilitated a system for ensuring good quality patient care, and organizations were expected to establish quality improvement programmes. These programmes included audit, clinical risk reduction programmes and processes that identified good practice as well as poor clinical performance. It was also anticipated that organizations would have procedures in place so that adverse events and patient complaints could be quickly identified, investigated, resolved, and lessons learned (Department of Health, 1997, 1998, 2000; WHO, 2005). Larizgoitia, Bouesseau, and Kelley (2013) highlight that whilst reporting of these adverse events has clearly had some impact on improving the quality of healthcare provision, not all organizations have implemented successful reporting processes and procedures. They posit that this might be because these organizations do not have a culture of patient safety, and that investigating these reports takes time which pressurized organizations may feel they do not have.

As chief executives had ultimate responsibility for ensuring services were of high quality, monthly and annual reports on clinical governance and the standards of quality of care achieved were to be submitted to Trust boards, ensuring that clinical governance was as high on the agenda as financial governance. Table 1.1 summarizes some of the key government White Papers and reports prior to a more in-depth discussion.

In order for clinical governance strategies to be successfully implemented, continuing professional development (CPD) became crucial for healthcare

Table 1.1 Government reports and organizations

The New NHS: Modern, Dependable (Department of Health, 1997)	The government's response to Allitt, Shipman, and the Bristol paediatric cardiac mortality rates Introduction of clinical governance that focused on improving the quality of healthcare
A First Class Service: Quality in the New NHS (Department of Health, 1998)	Outlined the government's strategy for ensuring quality care was provided to all
An Organisation with a Memory (Department of Health, 2000)	A report from an expert group on learning from adverse events in the NHS
High Quality Care for All: NHS Next Stage Review (Department of Health, 2008)	A review of the reforms since 1997 and 1998
NHS Five Year Forward View (NHS, 2014)	Outlined how NHS services needed to change
The NHS Long Term Plan (NHS, 2019)	Outlines the strategy for re-design of patient care within financial constraints, and for dealing with pressures placed on the workforce
National Institute for Clinical Excellence (NICE)	Launched in 1999 primarily to provide clinicians with evidence-based guidelines for the provision of care (National Service Frameworks). Lord Darzi recommended that the remit of NICE (now renamed National Institute for Health and Care Excellence) be increased to include the setting of independent standards (Department of Health, 2008)
Commission for Health Improvement (CHI)	Established in 1999. One of the key responsibilities of the CHI was to monitor and review local clinical governance provisions
Care Quality Commission (CQC)	Established in 2009 from the merger of the CHI, the Mental Health Act Commission, and the Commission for Social Care. Its remit is to ensure that national standards are met through monitoring and regulation of health and adult social care services in England

staff (CPD will be explored in more depth in Chapter 7). Staff were therefore expected to engage in professional development workshops which facilitated leadership skills as well as an understanding of the application of clinical governance strategies (Department of Health, 1997). It was also recognized that developments in technology and demographics were changing exponentially and therefore learning had to become lifelong and a continuous process (Sullivan and Garland, 2010). (Refer to Chapter 5, where education and training are discussed in more depth).

Clinical Governance Committees were established and Clinical Governance Leads appointed within UK hospital Trusts as a result of government directives. These individuals were senior clinicians who were to be responsible for ensuring that the necessary structures and processes were in place and their effectiveness continually monitored (Department of Health, 1998).

These Department of Health papers guaranteed that a number of national structures were established to ensure that quality of care was effective, efficient, and of a high standard. The two key organizations were:

- National Institute for Clinical Excellence (NICE)
- The Commission for Health Improvement (CHI)

National Institute for Clinical Excellence

NICE (now known as the National Institute for Health and Care Excellence) provides healthcare practitioners with specific evidence-based guidelines, including National Service Frameworks on a variety of conditions such as cancer care, children, chronic obstructive pulmonary disease, diabetes, coronary heart disease, older people, mental health, long-term conditions, and long-term neurological conditions.

The Commission for Health Improvement

One of the key responsibilities of the CHI was to monitor and review local clinical governance provisions and to support and provide advice on how to ameliorate and prevent adverse events (Department of Health, 1998, 2000).

The Prime Minister at the time, Gordon Brown, asked Lord Darzi, Junior Health Minister and a practising surgeon, to suggest a strategy to meet the health needs of Londoners. The report, *Healthcare for London: A Framework for Action*, was published in July 2007 (Department of Health, 2007). Darzi was also asked to review the reforms achieved since the Department of Health's 1997 and 1998 White Papers. Furthermore, he collaborated with patients and staff to identify a vision for the development and future of the health service in the twenty-first century. In his report *High Quality Care for All: NHS Next Stage Review*, Darzi envisioned that the UK would have "an NHS that gives patients and the public more information and choice, works in partnership and has quality of care at its heart" (Department of Health, 2008: 2).

Darzi recommended that the remit of NICE was to be increased to include the setting of more independent quality standards. Additionally, a new National Quality Board would give clear advice to ministers on the priority of those clinical standards. Key priorities focused on the provision of safe and effective quality care but also on ensuring that the patient's experience of care was good. This was endorsed by the Royal College of Nursing (RCN), which states on its website that the main focus of clinical governance is to improve the patient experience (Scrivener, 2010). Scrivener was an information manager on the RCN's quality improvement programme.

Care Quality Commission

In 2009, the Commission for Health Improvement, the Mental Health Act Commission, and the Commission for Social Care were amalgamated to become the Care Quality Commission (CQC). The key aim of the CQC is to ensure that national standards are met through monitoring and regulation of health and adult social care services in England. NHS organizations and social care providers now have to register with the CQC.

The CQC is a self-governing watchdog that audits and regulates establishments – namely hospitals, dentists, ambulances, care homes, and services in people's own homes and elsewhere – against a framework of standards to ensure that national standards of quality and safety are met. These standards include basic needs such as:

- Guaranteeing service users have the right food and liquids
- Making sure the environment is clean and safe
- Ensuring that patients and services users are involved in their own care, their dignity and respect are safeguarded, that staff have the required skills and knowledge, and that the quality of services is regularly audited (CQC, 2009)

More than 10 years later, the work of the CQC continues. In December 2018, the CQC published a report *Opening the Door to Change*. This report looked at aspects that led to Never Events, defined as "serious incidents that are wholly preventable because guidance or safety recommendations that provide strong systemic protective barriers are available at a national level and should have been implemented by all healthcare providers" (NHS Improvement, 2018: 4). The CQC reviewed policies and procedures across a range of acute and mental health Trusts. Fora, workshops, one-to-one interviews, and focus groups were undertaken with a range of providers and patient representatives. One of the key recommendations was the need for patient safety to become a priority. However, the CQC report clearly states that leaders responsible for patient safety should have the appropriate training in order to facilitate this drive. The need for the various regulators to standardize the governance processes and to have a standardized patient safety alert system was also identified (CQC, 2018).

Clinical Commissioning Groups

From April 2013, Clinical Commissioning Groups (CCGs) replaced Primary Care Trusts and one of their key aims was to meet patient needs through providing the "right care, right place, first time" (Department of Health, 2012a: 6). The NHS Commissioning Board also includes this statement in their vision for "ensuring we have the right staff, with the right skills in the right place" (Department of Health, 2012b: 22). It is evident that quality care remains on the national agenda, although recent events in 2012–2013 (Francis Report, 2013) suggest that there has been limited progress, since the phrase ensuring we have "the right staff with the right skills in the right place" (Department of Health, 2012a: 22) is a repetition of the phrase "doing the right things, at the right time, for the right people, and doing them right – first time" (Department of Health, 1997: 3.2).

By 2020, 135 CCGs had been established in England. For 2019–2020, these groups were responsible for approximately two-thirds of the total NHS England budget, which equates to approximately £80 billion (NHS Clinical Commissioners, 2020).

Key points

- The Department of Health is committed to improving the quality of healthcare
- Staff need to review practice continuously in order to meet national standards of care
- Clinical governance remains on the national agenda
- It is essential that leaders with a responsibility for patient safety have appropriate training to enable them to facilitate improvements in patient care

---

Defining clinical governance

Activity 1.1

Before reading the definitions below, write down four key words that you feel could be included in a definition of clinical governance. It will be interesting to see how your ideas link to the definitions.

The literature presents a number of definitions for us to consider. First,

A framework through which organisations are accountable for continuously improving the quality of services and safeguarding high standards of care by creating an environment in which clinical care will flourish. (Department of Health, 1998: 33)

According to Lugon (2005), healthcare professionals should incorporate clinical governance strategies into everyday practice, and one of the important things to note from the definition above (creating an environment) is that clinical governance is relevant to both staff and patients – therefore, the environment impacts on both staff and patients. For example, the quality of patient care could be affected if staff work in an environment in which support or opportunities to develop their knowledge and skills is lacking. Lack of resources (low staffing levels, equipment, and/or medication) could also impact on both staff and patients. From the patient's viewpoint, admission to a mixed ward could affect their overall experience and their perception of quality care.

A second definition to consider:

> Clinical Governance places a duty on all health professionals, clinicians and managers to ensure that the level of clinical service they deliver to patients is satisfactory, consistent and responsive. (Swage, 2004: 4)

Although cited in Swage (2004), the ideas for this definition stem from the Department of Health's 1997 White Paper, *The New NHS: Modern, Dependable*. This definition reinforces the need for all healthcare professionals, whether clinicians or managers, to be accountable for the service they provide to patients. Initially, the National Service Frameworks were one of the systems designed to support staff to do this; however, they have now been discontinued. Swage suggests that clinical governance is an "umbrella under which all aspects of quality can be continually monitored and it needs to be led by clinicians" (2004: 5).

A final definition to consider is that of Som (2004: 89):

> A governance system for healthcare organisations that promotes an integrated approach towards management of inputs, structures and processes to improve the outcome of the healthcare service delivery where health staff work in an environment of greater accountability for clinical quality.

One of the strengths of Som's definition is that it encapsulates and reinterprets the two Department of Health definitions, and in so doing captures the complexity of the issue. As well as considering the environment (Department of Health, 1998) and accountability (Swage, 2004), Som also addresses inputs, structure, processes, and outcome, each of which is aligned with clinical governance (Table 1.2). All of these concepts will be discussed and applied to practice in later chapters.

From the above definitions it is evident that all healthcare professionals have a responsibility to continuously develop practice and improve the quality of care provided and thus improve patient safety. However, for this to happen a blame culture needs to be avoided. According to Fetherston (2015), if staff are going to report near miss events, incident reporting forms need to be uncomplicated and staff need to be confident that their views and confidentiality will be respected. An all-embracing approach must be taken and all aspects of the event must be analysed, not just the final incident – that is, the last domino takes the blame (Ellahham, 2018). Furthermore, action plans need to be drawn up and most importantly communicated to all staff. Further education and training will likely also need to be provided (this will be discussed in more depth in Chapter 5).

Table 1.2   Attributes of clinical governance: Som's (2004) definitions

Inputs	Includes financial resources, human resources, infrastructure, and policy (where quality is a legislative requirement of the organization)
Structure	Includes the requirement to provide education and training and continuing professional development, and guidelines for clinical care, for example integrated care pathways, clinical risk management, promoting evidence-based medicine, audit and leadership development. CEOs to be accountable for the standard of care provided
Processes	Includes the implementation of risk management, education and training, leadership development, audit, and management of patient information (confidentiality and anonymity). It also includes processes to record near misses and adverse events
Outcomes	Includes continuous quality improvements (CQI), patient satisfaction, and reduced number of "near misses" and adverse events. Better rapport between patients and clinicians and improved collaboration between professionals and managers are also stressed. Additionally, interventions being supported through evidence-based practice are included (discussed further in Chapter 7)

Activity 1.2

- Have another look at the four key words you wrote down at the beginning of this section. Have they changed and, if so, why?
- Which is your preferred definition?
- Why do you prefer one definition over the others?

Using Som's four organizational dimensions (see Figure 1.3), analyse the incidents discussed at the beginning of this chapter to see where the problems arose in relation to inputs, structure, processes, and outcome. The questions below will help to guide your thinking:

Inputs

– Did financial, human, or environmental resources lead to the incident?

Structure

- Was a clear education and training programme available?
- Were guidelines for clinical care evident?
- Was there a failure with leadership?

Processes

- What processes were in place? Risk management? Leadership development? Implementation of education and training and the recording of near misses and adverse events?

Outcome

- How did the above impact on the outcome? For example, continuous quality improvement (CQI), improved patient satisfaction, better communication and collaboration, and reduced number of near misses?

Figure 1.3 Four organizational dimensions

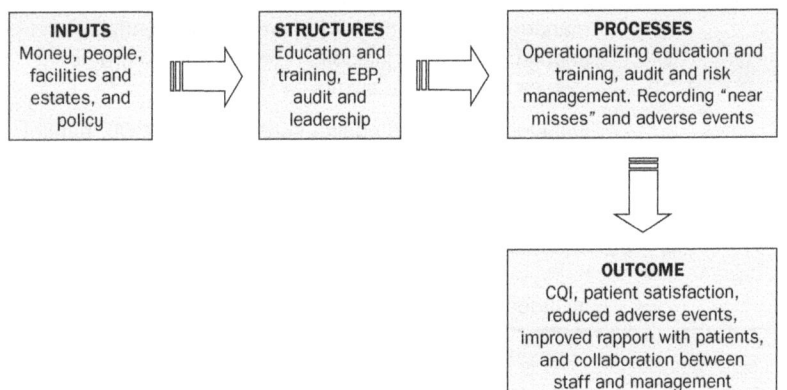

Adapted from: Som (2004).

The framework of clinical governance

The definition of clinical governance presented by the Department of Health (1998) states that clinical governance is a framework, and, as previously discussed, Swage says that clinical governance "provides an umbrella under which all aspects of quality can be gathered and continuously monitored" (2004: 5), but what does this actually involve? Figure 1.4 illustrates this more clearly. Clinical governance is the overarching framework and can be implemented through each strategy on the spokes of this umbrella. It can be seen that some of the spokes link to Som's organizational dimensions out-lined above.

Braithwaite and Travaglia (2008) and Buja *et al.* (2018) suggest that further aspects need to be added to achieve a successful clinical governance frame-work. Braithwaite and Travaglia suggest that there is also "a need for organi-sations to have vigilant governing boards and bodies and a need for there to be a focus on ethics and regulating qualified privilege" (2008: 12). Focusing on primary care, Buja *et al.* (2018) sought to design a clinical governance frame-work to improve the quality of care of chronic diseases by bringing together all activities for every patient episode of care, be they administrative, support, or clinical services. They stated that every interaction with patients and their fam-ilies should focus on their values within a fully integrated service which is accountable to patients and society. Best clinical governance practices should be at the core, including quality assurance, risk management, technology assessment, patient satisfaction, patient empowerment, and patient engage-ment. In order to achieve this, there is a requirement to carry out a population health needs assessment, ensuring that healthcare interventions are evidence-based, all professionals working within the practice are obliged to engage with continuing professional development and education, and there is a strong focus on team-building and communication.

The strategies discussed in later chapters will be aligned to the umbrella and Som's (2004) organizational dimensions.

Figure 1.4 The framework of clinical governance

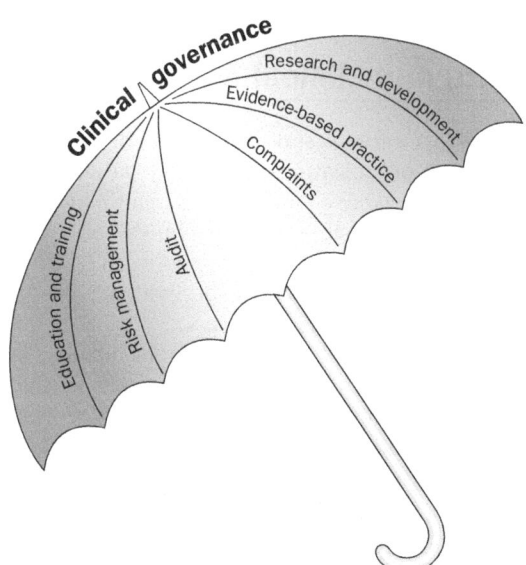

Defining quality

Quality is a personal construct dependent on one's beliefs and values and therefore quality could be considered to link to one's perception. Moullin (2003: 13) defines quality succinctly as "fitness for purpose" but one could then question what this means. If each organization sets its own standards and purpose, then it could be perceived that the quality of care would vary and the impact of this could be that quality of care could be poor in some organizations. Ovretveit provides a more in-depth definition: "Fully meeting the needs of those who need the service most, at the lowest cost to the organisation, within the limits and directives set by higher authorities" (1990, cited in Moullin, 2003: 14).

For Darzi, quality can be defined as "clinically effective, personal and safe" (Department of Health, 2008: 8–9), while Birnbaum and Van Buren view it as a "journey not a destination" (2010: 81). This last definition is a useful one for organizations because in order to arrive at successful outcomes, quality must continuously be improved through constantly developing inputs, structure, and processes (Som, 2004).

Whatever definition of quality is used, there needs to be an understanding between the organization and service users, carers, and the public.

Linking quality and clinical governance

Quality is of interest to various stakeholders, both internal and external to health and social care organizations, including patients, relatives, hospital staff, and government. They have an interest in healthcare, they deliver healthcare, and/or are held responsible for the clinical effectiveness of service delivery. Clinical governance aims to put the delivery of clinical quality at the centre of healthcare provision. It should be evidence-based, widely shared, using skilled staff and appropriate facilities.

As suggested by Som (2004), clinical governance includes implementing evidence-based practice into everyday patient care to ensure that healthcare professionals know what they are doing works and why it works (see Figure 1.5). It includes continuous quality improvement so that healthcare professionals always aim to improve practice, guarantee that risks are managed, and lessons learned from incidents and accidents are shared. Shared learning (education and training) ensures that healthcare professionals aim to prevent what mistakes they can, limit what they cannot prevent and, most importantly, learn from mistakes that are made and to prevent them happening again in the future. Finally, clinical governance includes clinical audit to assess and evaluate compliance, to encourage reflection on individual and team work while checking to see if what should happen is indeed happening.

Figure 1.5 Linking quality and clinical governance

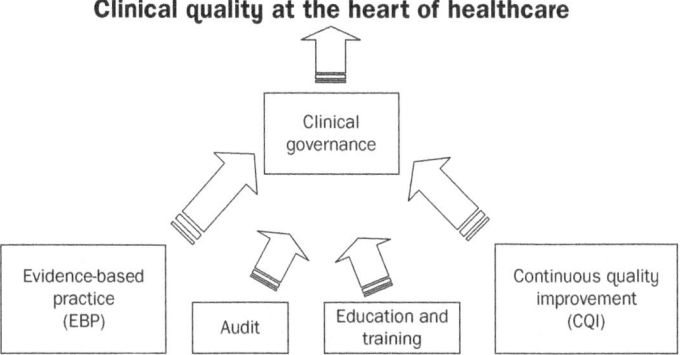

Engagement of patients/service users

The birth of patient/service user engagement

Since its inception in 1948, the NHS has changed and continues to change, and after the high-profile cases discussed earlier it became essential to re-establish trust in the NHS. The NHS is funded through public taxation and therefore service users, carers, and the general public are in the main interested in the standard of care provided. These groups increasingly want to be given the opportunity to be involved and have a say in how healthcare services are developed in the future (Haxby, Hunter, and Jaggar, 2010). In addition, ready access to the internet has enabled service users to become more knowledgeable about their health and therefore what they expect a healthcare service to provide. Lord Darzi strongly acknowledged the importance of putting service users at the centre of healthcare (Department of Health, 2008). Following the Darzi Report, service users began to be involved in decision-making in relation to where they received their care package – for example, in which hospital they wished to receive secondary care – and the level of care they could expect. This involvement of service users in decision-making has helped to reduce medical paternalism.

Definitions of patient/service user engagement

According to Matthews (2010: 314) service user involvement is defined as:

> *individual involvement (for example, the central role of patients in decisions about their own health and care) and involvement at a more collective level (patient representatives, for example actively contributing to NHS policy and planning decisions).*

Instead of service user involvement, the Care Quality Commission uses the term patient and public engagement. The CQC runs an Acting Together programme within England, which involves discussions with experts by experience, that is, those who have first-hand experience of health and social care services thus ensuring that the voices of service users are heard. These experts are very much part of the CQC in that they are part of the inspections that take place, and they are also included in process development activities within the CQC. During the unannounced visits, the CQC provide the experts with topics they would like discussed, enabling the experts to talk independently with residents in care homes and/or patients in hospitals to elicit their viewpoints on what organizations are doing well and what could be improved upon. Any concerns are then reported back to the CQC inspector.

Rationale for engagement

One of the key reasons for engaging service users and carers is because, as the recipients of care, they have an understanding of specific interventions. Ultimately, they are experienced and have ideas on how a service needs to be developed to ensure continuous quality improvement. Healthcare professionals may feel that their knowledge and expertise are being challenged (medical paternalism), but gaining an understanding of the service user's perspective will benefit future provision and improve patient care.

Redesign versus co-design

Bate and Robert go further and state that the above is not enough: "The role of users and the value and justification for their being there is to bring the knowledge of their experience to the table so that the designers can work with them to translate and build that knowledge into new and future designs" (2007: 27). These authors conclude that rather than redesigning the system around the patient, the service could be co-designed with the patient. This is further supported by Frank Gehry (2003), who states that "without the client, you're one hand, you're the sound of one hand clapping. The client is the variable, and if the client engages with you, that's the opportunity" (cited in Bate and Robert, 2007: 16). Although Gehry is speaking from an architectural perspective, his thoughts echo those of Bate and Robert.

Level of engagement

Following the Darzi Report (Department of Health, 2008), it is now widely agreed that service users need to be involved and engaged at a variety of levels within healthcare organizations, including at board level, committee level, and at an individual level (Bond and Magill, 2010). This involvement has led to the need for increased communication and greater collaboration, so that service users can have a positive impact on decisions and their presence is not simply tokenistic. This could be seen as "adding value" both to professionals and to service users (Bond and Magill, 2010).

Organizations must ensure that the improvement of quality care is continuous (continuous quality improvement) and, as Matthews (2010) highlights, this also means that service users must be engaged in constant discussions and plans. In other words, their involvement is not a single event. Whilst healthcare professionals have an understanding of the evidence base of care, it is the recipients who have an understanding of the experience and so through working together there is a better chance of standards, as set out by NICE, being raised and the expectations of both the professionals and service users being met.

Example of good practice – Together: For Mental Wellbeing

In 2012, NICE established a shared learning database. Together: For Mental Wellbeing is an organization that established some training sessions designed, delivered, and evaluated by those who used mental health services. The key aim of these learning sessions was to inform those working within mental health services about service user involvement so that staff could make positive changes to their practice. Sessions were developed to give health and social care practitioners an understanding of the lived experience of mental health service users. They also helped practitioners to gain an understanding of what worked well and what did not work, from the service user's perspective. Lastly, suggestions were made on how practice could be developed and improved further (NICE, 2012).

Activity 1.3

Access the following links to gain an understanding of strategies that aim to develop service user engagement within mental health:

– Barnet, Enfield and Haringey Mental Health Trust

  https://www.beh-mht.nhs.uk/news/new-service-user-involvement-and-en-gagement-strategy/553 (accessed: 7 March 2021)

– Greater Manchester Mental Health NHS Foundation Trust

  https://www.gmmh.nhs.uk/download.cfm?doc=docm93jijm4n4373 (accessed: 7 March 2021)

– The King's Fund

  https://www.kingsfund.org.uk/topics/patient-involvement?gclid=EAIaI-QobChMIrNChqKnQ7gIVAbDtCh1GbgtSEAAYASAAEgIC-vD_BwE (accessed: 7 March 2021)

Key point

Service users and their families need to be involved in planning and evaluating their care.

> ### Activity 1.4
>
> - How are service users included in the delivery of their care in your workplace?
> - Thinking about your workplace and Bate and Robert's (2007) suggestion, are service users involved in redesigning the service around the patient or co-designing the service with the patient? If the former, how might this be changed?
> - The King's Fund is an independent charitable organization involved with improving the quality of healthcare in England. This includes working with the public and patients in service design. The following link will facilitate your learning further:
>   - https://www.kingsfund.org.uk/topics/patient-involvement?gclid= EAIaIQobChMIrNChqKnQ7gIVAbDtCh1GbgtSEAAYASAAEgIC-vD_BwE (accessed: 7 March 2021)

Practice examples

Another aspect to consider is that the service user's priorities may differ from those of the professional.

This is illustrated in the early career of M.G. as an occupational therapist, working on a stroke rehabilitation ward. As an occupational therapist, a priority of mine was to facilitate patients to be able to dress themselves independently. One of my patients explained to me that although they could get dressed without any assistance, it would take hours and leave them exhausted, so they would prefer to employ someone to dress them. By paying someone, it enabled this patient to spend their time engaged more purposively in their hobbies. This illustrates how my priorities were different from those of the patient.

Bond and Magill (2010) identify other examples where priorities between the professional and service user differ. First, an individual whose hobby was fishing prioritized resolving his incontinence problem first before other multiple problems. By having his incontinence problem resolved, it meant he could spend the day fishing without any embarrassments.

Secondly, a Muslim patient wished to have the osteoarthritis in his knees dealt with prior to other problems, to enable him to kneel to pray. This person spent a number of hours each week praying in the local mosque and being able to kneel without pain had become the main priority.

These examples illustrate how service users can and should be involved at a micro or personal level with co-designing their healthcare. Bate and Robert (2007) would take this further to empower service users to co-design the service at a macro level.

Having discussed the importance of establishing relationships and partnerships between service users and healthcare providers, it is important to consider how service users can be involved.

Methods of engagement

> ### Activity 1.5
>
> Write a list of the different methods that could be used to involve service users in planning and co-designing healthcare services in your own area of practice.

Some suggestions are provided below, which might be similar to the ones you identified in your answer to the above activity. Chapter 3 will discuss another process that could be used through setting up quality circles.

Service users/experts by experience can also become involved with clinical governance through surveys distributed to gain an understanding of their perceptions. Surveys collect quantitative data, for example through using Likert scales. For a more in-depth understanding, qualitative methods could be used, such as one-to-one interviews. However, this could be a daunting experience for the service user who might see the professional as someone in a position of power and therefore they may feel intimidated and not want to give their true opinion. One way to overcome this is to engage service users/experts by experience in focus groups. One advantage of focus groups is that a number of individuals (6–8) can be involved in discussions at the same time, thus making them more comfortable about sharing their opinions (Sale, 2005; Wright and Hill, 2003).

Patient Voices Programme

This programme offers service users/patients a very different opportunity from the above method of using surveys and interviews. One of the key aims of the Patient Voices Programme is to put patients at the heart of healthcare (Department of Health, 2008) to facilitate collaboration between healthcare professionals and patients to work together to continue to develop patient care. Initially, Patient Voices was funded by the NHS Clinical Governance Support Team (Patient Voices Programme) and they have been sharing stories from patients since 2003.

Patient Voices are short digital stories using a variety of media, such as video and audio recordings or music. These stories allow individuals to share their experiences and feelings on what it was like to be the recipient of healthcare. These stories are shared with hospital Trust boards and teams. As well as providing examples of excellent care, digital stories could provide a number of examples of poor care, such as near misses, poor access to care, or negative staff attitudes.

Evidence from Manchester Mental Healthcare Trust shows that these stories enable strategy planners and frontline staff to practise in a more informed and compassionate manner and, as a result, complaints in relation to care and staff attitudes have fallen.

Key point

The Patient Voices Programme encourages partnership working between healthcare professionals and service users and could be deemed to be less frightening and more productive than interviews or questionnaires. See:

https://www.patientvoices.org.uk/who-we-are/about-patient-voices (accessed: 7 March 2021)

Key points summary

In this chapter, we have considered the historical perspective and the clinical issues that led to the inception of the concept of organizational clinical governance. Clinical governance is an overarching framework under which various structures and processes sit (Som, 2004), thereby ensuring that the quality of healthcare is continuously improved.

Collaboration and partnership working between health and social care staff and the service users/experts by experience who have first-hand experience of healthcare are recommended. Also recommended is the notion of involving service users/experts by experience in co-design of the service rather than redesign of their care (Bate and Robert, 2007).

- Clinical governance is a framework used to improve the quality of care provided
- Clinical governance relates to both staff and service users
- All staff employed within health and social care are accountable for the standards of care provided
- For quality care provision to be successful, patient and public engagement in service evaluation and development and therefore involvement is essential

Implications for practice

- Healthcare organizations must ensure that all healthcare staff, service users, and members of the public are involved in the development of the quality of care
- Shared learning and candour should be part of an organization's ethos
- A shared leadership approach supports clinical governance

- Two-way communication is essential to minimize adverse clinical incidents
- Continuing professional development is essential for all health and social care practitioners

End-of-chapter questions

1 How does an understanding of the definitions of clinical governance help you develop your practice?
2 Knowing that clinical governance is everyone's responsibility, how could you become more proactive in implementing your organization's strategy for quality improvement?
3 What is the role of the clinical governance lead in your organization?
4 How do you feed into this role?

See the Appendix on page 253 for suggested answers to these questions.

References

Bate, P. and Robert, G. (2007) *Bringing User Experience to Healthcare Improvement: The concepts, methods and practices of experience-based design.* Oxford: Radcliffe Publishing.

Birnbaum, D. and Van Buren, J. (2010) Applying continuous improvement in public reporting: What should government reports do for quality improvement?, *Clinical Governance: An International Journal,* 15 (2): 79–91.

Bond, J. and Magill, J. (2010) Patient and public consultation, in E. Haxby, D. Hunter, and S. Jaggar (eds.) *An Introduction to Clinical Governance and Patient Safety.* Oxford: Oxford University Press.

Braithwaite, J. and Travaglia, J. (2008) An overview of clinical governance policies, practices and initiatives, *Australian Health Review,* 32 (1): 10–22.

Bristol Royal Infirmary Inquiry (2001) *The Report of the Public Inquiry into Children's Heart Surgery at the Bristol Royal Infirmary 1984–1995: Learning from Bristol.* Bristol: Bristol Royal Infirmary Inquiry.

Buja, A., Toffanin, R., Claus, M., Ricciardi, W., Damiani, G., Baldo, V. *et al.* (2018) Developing a new clinical governance framework for chronic disease in primary care: An umbrella review, *BMJ Open,* 8 (7): e020626. Available at: https://doi.org/10.1136/bmjopen-2017-020626.

Care Quality Commission (CQC) (2009) *Care Quality Commission (Registration) Regulations 2009.* Available at: https://www.cqc.org.uk/files/care-quality-commission-registration-regulations-2009 (accessed: 7 March 2021).

Care Quality Commission (CQC) (2017) *The State of Care in Mental Health Services 2014 to 2017.* Available at: https://www.cqc.org.uk/publications/major-report/state-care-mental-health-services-2014-2017 (accessed: 7 March 2021).

Care Quality Commission (CQC) (2018) *Opening the Door to Change: NHS safety culture and the need for transformation.* Available at: https://www.cqc.org.uk/publications/themed-work/opening-door-change (accessed: 25 June 2021).

Clothier Report (1994) *The Allitt Inquiry: Independent inquiry relating to deaths and injuries on the children's ward at Grantham and Kesteven General Hospital (The Clothier Report).* London: HMSO.

Department of Health (1997) *The New NHS: Modern, Dependable.* Available at: https://www.gov.uk/government/publications/the-new-nhs (accessed: 7 March 2021).

Department of Health (1998) *A First Class Service: Quality in the new NHS.* London: Department of Health.

Department of Health (2000) *An Organisation with a Memory.* London: HMSO.

Department of Health (2006) *Good Doctors, Safer Patients: Proposals to strengthen the system to assure and improve the performance of doctors and to protect the safety of patients.* London: Department of Health.

Department of Health (2007) *Healthcare for London: A framework for action.* London: Department of Health.

Department of Health (2008) *High Quality Care for All: NHS next stage review final report.* London: HMSO. Available at: http://www.official-documents.gov.uk/document/cm74/7432/7432.pdf (accessed: 7 March 2021).

Department of Health (2012a) *An Organisation with a Memory.* London: HMSO.

Department of Health (2012b) *Compassion in Practice: Nursing, midwifery and care staff. Our vision and strategy.* London: HMSO. Available at: https://www.england.nhs.uk/wp-content/uploads/2012/12/compassion-in-practice.pdf (accessed 25 June 2021).

Department of Health (2012c) *Transforming Care: A national response to Winterbourne View Hospital – Department of Health Review: Final report.* Available at: https://assets.publishing.service.gov.uk/government/uploads/system/uploads/attachment_data/file/213215/final-report.pdf (accessed: 7 March 2021).

Ellahham, S. (2018) The domino effect of medical errors, *American Journal of Medical Quality*, 34 (4): 412–413.

Fetherston, T. (2015) The importance of critical incident reporting – and how to do it, *Community Eye Health Journal*, 28 (90): 26–27.

Francis Report (2013) *Report of the Mid Staffordshire NHS Foundation Trust Public Inquiry.* London: HMSO.

Gehry, F. (2003) *Gehry Talks: Architecture and process.* London: Thames & Hudson.

Haxby, E., Hunter, D.H., and Jaggar, S. (eds.) (2010) *An Introduction to Clinical Governance and Patient Safety.* Oxford: Oxford University Press.

Healthcare Commission (2007) *Investigation into Outbreaks of Clostridium difficile at Maidstone and Tunbridge Wells NHS Trust.* London: Commission for Healthcare Audit.

Henderson, J., Gao, H., and Redshaw, M. (2013) Experiencing maternity care: The care received and perceptions of women from different ethnic groups, *BMC Pregnancy and Childbirth*, 13: 196. Available at: https://doi.org/10.1186/1471-2393-13-196.

Larzigoitia, I., Bouesseau, M.-C., and Kelley, E. (2013) WHO efforts to promote reporting adverse events and global learning, *Journal of Public Health Research*, 2 (3): e29. Available at: https://doi.org/10.4081/jphr.2013.e29.

Lugon, M. (2005) Clinical governance – from rhetoric to reality, *Current Paediatrics*, 15 (6): 460–465.

MacDonald, A. (1996) Responding to the results of the Beverly Allitt inquiry, *Nursing Times*, Jan 10–6:92 (2): 23–25.

Matthews, R. (2010) Patient and public involvement (PPI), in E. Haxby, D. Hunter, and S. Jaggar (eds.) *An Introduction to Clinical Governance and Patient Safety.* Oxford: Oxford University Press.

Moullin, M. (2003) *Delivering Excellence in Health and Social Care.* Maidenhead: Open University Press.

NHS (2014) *Five Year Forward View.* Available at: https://www.england.nhs.uk/wp-content/uploads/2014/10/5yfv-web.pdf (accessed: 7 March 2012).

NHS (2017) *Next Steps on the Five Year Forward View.* Available at: https://www.england.nhs.uk/wp-content/uploads/2017/03/NEXT-STEPS-ON-THE-NHS-FIVE-YEAR-FORWARD-VIEW.pdf (accessed: 7 March 2021).

NHS (2019) *The NHS Long Term Plan.* Available at: https://www.longtermplan.nhs.uk/publication/nhs-long-term-plan/ (accessed: 7 March 2021).

NHS Clinical Commissioners (2020) *The Independent Collective Voice of Clinical Commissioners.* Available at: https://www.nhscc.org/ccgs (accessed: 7 March 2021).

NHS Improvement (2018) *Never Events Policy and Framework.* Available at: https://www.england.nhs.uk/wp-content/uploads/2020/11/Revised-Never-Events-policy-and-framework-FINAL.pdf (accessed: 7 March 2021).

NHS Resolution (2020) *Annual Report and Accounts* 2019/20. London: HMSO. Available at: https://resolution.nhs.uk/2020/07/16/nhs-resolutions-annual-report-and-accounts-2019-20/.

NICE (2012) *Good Practice in Service User Involvement Training.* Available at: https://www.nice.org.uk/sharedlearning/good-practice-in-service-user-involvement-training (accessed: 7 March 2021).

Ockenden Report (2020) *Maternity Services at the Shrewsbury and Telford Hospital NHS Trust.* Available at: https://assets.publishing.service.gov.uk/government/uploads/system/uploads/attachment_data/file/943011/Independent_review_of_maternity_services_at_Shrewsbury_and_Telford_Hospital_NHS_Trust.pdf (accessed: 7 March 2021).

Sale, D. (2005) *Understanding Clinical Governance and Quality Assurance: Making it happen.* Basingstoke: Palgrave Macmillan.

Scrivener, R. (2010) Nursing practice issues. Available at: http://www.rcn.org.uk (accessed: 7 March 2021).

Slawomirski, L., Auraaen, A., and Klazinga, N.S. (2017) *The Economics of Patient Safety: Strengthening a value-based approach to reducing patient harm at a national level.* No. 96: Paris: OECD Publishing. Available at: https://doi.org/10.1787/5a9858cd-en.

Smith, Dame J. (2002) *The Shipman Inquiry: Death certification and the investigation of deaths by coroners.* Manchester: HMSO.

Som, C. (2004) Clinical governance: A fresh look at its definition, *Clinical Governance: An International Journal*, 9 (2): 87–90.

Sullivan, E. and Garland, G. (2010) *Practical Leadership and Management in Healthcare: For nurses and allied health professionals.* London: Pearson.

Swage, T. (2004) *Clinical Governance in Healthcare Practice.* London: Butterworth-Heinemann.

World Health Organization (WHO) (2005) *World Alliance for Patient Safety. WHO draft guidelines for adverse event reporting and learning systems: From information to action.* Available at: https://apps.who.int/iris/handle/10665/69797 (accessed: 7 March 2021).

World Health Organization (WHO) (2017) *Medication Without Harm: Global patient safety challenge on medication safety.* Geneva: WHO. Available at: http://apps.who.int/iris/bitstream/handle/10665/255263/WHO-HIS-SDS-2017.6-eng.pdf?sequence=1 (accessed: 25 June 2021).

World Health Organization (WHO) (2019) *World Health Statistics: Monitoring health for the SDGs.* Available at: https://www.who.int/publications/i/item/world-health-statistics-2019-monitoring-health-for-the-sdgs-sustainable-development-goals (accessed: 7 March 2021).

Wright, J. and Hill, P. (2003) *Clinical Governance.* London: Churchill Livingstone.

2 Quality: the key issues

Gail E. Lansdown

Learning objectives

By the end of this chapter, the reader will have a better understanding of:

- The global push for improving the delivery of quality healthcare
- The reporting of Never Events and Sentinel Events
- The incidence, morbidity, and mortality of a number of quality issues that impact on patient/client care

Introduction

The previous chapter introduced the concept of clinical governance and its importance in ensuring that standards and quality patient care are continuously monitored and improved. This chapter will focus on the incidence and mortality of eight quality issues that impact on patients/service users both locally and internationally. These examples have been taken from a variety of settings – acute, community, and mental health services. The following chapters will explore the causes of these quality issues and will discuss clinical governance strategies that can be used to improve quality care.

The examples discussed in this chapter are taken from students' assignments and, whilst the incidents might not fall in NHS Improvement (2018) or The Joint Commission's (2020) top ten reported Sentinel Events, they illustrate incidents that occur regularly in practice and demonstrate how the clinical governance framework may well not have been appropriately implemented by all staff.

Never Events and Sentinel Events

"Never Events are defined as serious incidents that are wholly preventable because guidance or safety recommendations that provide strong systemic protective barriers are available at a national level and should have been implemented by all healthcare providers" (NHS Improvement, 2018: 4). A Sentinel Event is defined by American healthcare accreditation organization The Joint Commission (2020), as any unanticipated event in a healthcare setting resulting in death or serious physical or psychological injury to a patient or patients, not related to the natural course of the patient's illness.

The UK is one of the few countries to publish data on Never Events. The Never Events policy and framework was revised in 2018. A Never Event is of great concern because the implication is that the safety of patients has been compromised (NHS, 2018). It must be said that having a list of Never Events is not to assign blame and reinforce a blame culture within the organization, but to identify the importance of learning from the event occurring in the first place and making sure it does not occur again. Learning from the error is key and changing practice can only improve patient safety. To this end, the Care Quality Commission in the UK is working with NHS Improvement to identify what can be done to ensure Never Events do not occur (NHS, 2018).

Incident reporting systems are not new in healthcare and each country will have its own documentation. The UK has a reporting system for Never Events, namely the Strategic Executive Information System (StEIS) (NHS, 2018). The Joint Commission (2020) collects data on Sentinel Events in the USA. The Hong Kong Hospital Authority also has a reporting system, the Adverse Incident Reporting System (AIRS), with the Hospital Authority issuing an annual report on sentinel and serious untoward events (Hospital Authority Hong Kong, 2021). For each event, organizations must scrutinize what happened, why it happened, where it happened, and when it happened.

Of 250 incidents that occurred between April and November 2020 in the UK, 226 were deemed to be Never Events (NHS, 2020). Adverse events and near misses should also be prevented and staff within healthcare must report any event or near miss. Examples of a near miss include a missed diagnosis, a missed referral, the incorrect use of hoists, or the incorrect use of moving and handling techniques; the latter two examples could lead to a patient falling.

Never Events reported in 2020 fell into the following categories:

- Wrong site surgery
- Retained foreign object post procedure
- Misplaced naso- or orogastric tubes and feed administered
- Wrong implant/prosthesis
- Unintentional connection of a patient requiring oxygen to an air flowmeter
- Administration of medication by wrong route
- Transfusion or transplantation of ABO incompatible blood components or organs
- Overdose of insulin due to abbreviations or incorrect device
- Failure to instal functional collapsible shower or curtain rails
- Scalding of patients
- Mis-selection of a strong potassium solution
- Mis-selection of high-strength midazolam during conscious sedation
- Chest or neck entrapment in bedrails

In the NHS Never Event Report (NHS, 2021), the events are listed by healthcare provider.

In the United States, The Joint Commission (2020) collects data on Sentinel Events, with 844 events being reported in 2019 that fell into the following categories:

- Care management: falls, delays in treatment, medication management
- Surgical or invasive procedures: unintended retention of a foreign object, wrong site, operative/post-operative complications
- Suicide: off-site within 72 hours, inpatient, Emergency Department
- Protection: self-harm, assault, infant abduction
- Environment: fire, medical equipment, medical/surgical supplies
- Product or device: medication equipment, medical/surgical supplies
- Unassigned events at the time of the report

Whilst events are discussed in some detail in The Joint Commission annual reports (e.g. 2020), and bar charts are given to show numbers of events from 2005 to date, healthcare providers are not named. The Joint Commission also states that commonly reported Sentinel Events remained similar in recent years but identified suicide and fall reductions as priorities for 2020.

The Hong Kong Hospital Authority (Hospital Authority Hong Kong, 2021) collects data on Sentinel Events and Serious Untoward Events. During the period October 2019 to September 2020, 24 Sentinel Events and 50 Serious Untoward Events were reported. The categories were as follows:

Sentinel Events

- Surgical error, wrong patient/part
- Retained instruments/material

- ABO blood incompatibility
- Medication error resulting in permanent loss of function or death
- Gas embolism
- Inpatient suicide
- Maternal morbidity
- Wrong infant/abduction
- Other adverse events resulting in permanent loss of function or death

Serious Untoward Events

- Medication error which could have resulted in death or permanent harm
- Patient misidentification

It is interesting to note the difference in Never Events in the UK and Sentinel Events in the USA and Hong Kong. It should also be remembered that the reporting of most Sentinel Events in the USA is voluntary and probably only represents a small proportion of the true number. Conversely, in the UK, Never Events must be reported.

Activity 2.1

If you are not familiar with the UK's list of Never Events, access the link below:
    https://webarchive.nationalarchives.gov.uk/20200501112015/https://improvement.nhs.uk/documents/2899/Never_Events_list_2018_FINAL_v7.pdf (accessed: 7 March 2021)

- Does the country where you work identify Never Events such as those listed in the link above?
- Think about your practice as a health/social care professional and list some examples of Never Events, adverse events, errors, and near misses that you have come across.
- Were these reported and, if not, why not?
- Do you know where and how to access the specific forms for reporting?

The following events, whilst not necessarily included in the three lists above, are events encountered by our students in the UK and Hong Kong.

Needle stick and sharps injuries

Needle stick and sharps injuries (NSSIs) occur around the globe, across all staff working within a healthcare environment, and in all settings where needles and sharps are used. NSSIs are considered among the most widespread occupational accidents in hospitals (Ochmann and Wicker, 2020). Even when standard precautions are observed, NSSIs are common (King and Strony, 2019).

Moreover, NSSIs have had a negative effect on the physical and mental health and wellbeing of millions of healthcare workers over the past decades (King and Strony, 2019). Despite the numbers of NSSIs having fallen over the past 30 years, they still do occur on a frequent basis, even when guidelines are in place (Cooke and Stephens, 2017).

In a systematic review and meta-analysis of the global prevalence and device-related causes of NSSIs, Bouya *et al.* (2020) stated that more than 2 million occupational NSSIs among 35 million healthcare workers occur every year (WHO, 2019). Groneberg *et al.* (2020), using the New Quality and Quantity Indices in Science platform, analysed 2,987 research articles from around the world and found that although 106 countries participated in research into NSSIs, swathes of Africa and South America did not. The authors believe that the WHO's (2019) global estimate of 2 million NSSIs annually is likely to be an underestimation due to patchy reporting.

Healthcare workers who experience an NSSI are at risk of contracting a number of infectious diseases, including hepatitis B, hepatitis C, and HIV. Globally, 39% of healthcare workers with hepatitis C, 37% of healthcare workers with hepatitis B, and 4.4% of healthcare workers with HIV were infected as a result of a sharps injuries (Cooke and Stephens, 2017).

Accessing articles from PubMed, Web of Science, and Scopus, Cooke and Stephens (2017) analysed the findings from 87 studies in which 50,916 healthcare workers from 31 countries took part. Despite existing strategies, they concluded that management strategies were lacking and/or there was a lack of compliance with available procedures. To reduce the risk of NSSIs, they suggest the following:

- Ensuring standard precautions are applied
- Regular training on prevention and correct recapping
- A robust NSSI reporting system
- Encouraging staff to report NSSIs
- Ensuring policies across all areas are clear and uniform
- The implementation of guidelines should be monitored regularly by an infection control committee
- Regular verbal and practical tests should be undertaken by healthcare staff on knowledge, attitudes, and performance regarding standard precautions

COVID-19 and NSSIs

Some studies have reported SARS-CoV-2 RNA in either plasma or serum, and the virus can replicate in blood cells. However, the role of bloodborne transmission remains uncertain and transmission through this route may be low (Chang *et al.*, 2020; Wang *et al.*, 2020).

Psychological impact of NSSIs

The humanistic, clinical, and economic burden for healthcare workers post NSSI is significant, with staff suffering from psychological stress and direct and indirect costs impacting the organization (Cooke and Stephens, 2017).

Activity 2.2

- Have you had, or do you know someone who has had, a needle stick or sharps injury?
- How did the injury occur?
- Was the injury reported?
- What was the outcome of the injury? Was treatment required? Was time taken off from work?
- Has there been a psychological impact?
- Were standard precautions followed?

Hospital-acquired infections

Hospitals, nursing homes, and outpatient departments are places where the acquisition of a hospital-acquired infection (HAI) is more likely. Until the advent of COVID-19, the most common types of HAI, or nosocomial infection, were surgical wound infection, respiratory infection, genitourinary infection, and gastrointestinal infection. The immunocompromised, the elderly, and young children are usually the most susceptible and infections are transmitted from hospital staff, poor infection control procedures, or droplets from other infected patients. HAIs are common, costly (directly, indirectly, and intangibly), and potentially lethal (Krein et al., 2011).

Methicillin-resistant *Staphylococcus aureus*

The haphazard use of antibiotics contributed to the advent of drug-resistant bacteria, such as methicillin-resistant *Staphylococcus aureus* (MRSA) (Thorat et al., 2021). Whilst not always life-threatening, MRSA is a global cause of increased treatment costs, increased length of stay, and risk of death.

Methicillin was first used in 1959 to treat infections caused by penicillin-resistant *Staphylococcus aureus*, and two years later, in 1961, reports from the UK suggested that *S. aureus* isolates had become resistant to methicillin (Enright et al., 2002). MRSA has a serious financial impact on patients and hospitals (Hudson et al., 2011), and until the 1990s MRSA mainly infected people who regularly attended healthcare facilities (healthcare-associated MRSA or HA-MRSA). Hudson et al. (2011) state that the rate of HA-MRSA (symptomatic and asymptomatic) in general hospital populations in the United States is 6–21%, with 9–24% infections in intensive care units (ICUs).

Since the 1990s, however, community-associated MRSA (CA-MRSA) has become more prevalent and causes infection in young children and adults who have not had previous contact with healthcare facilities. CA-MRSA has been reported globally (Wallin, Hern, and Frazee, 2008), and it is particularly virulent in young children. Some reports suggest that CA-MRSA is becoming more prevalent than HA-MRSA in some hospital settings (D'Agata *et al.*, 2009; Popovich *et al.*, 2013). In 2017 in the United States, an estimated 119,247 *S. aureus* infections were believed to have occurred, with 19,832 associated deaths (Kourtis *et al.*, 2019). Kourtis *et al.* state that, despite reductions in MRSA since 2005, community-based infections declined less markedly – indeed, they increased slightly from 2012 to 2017.

Research undertaken by Mao *et al.* (2019) indicated that patients with central venous catheters, sputum suction, and total hospital stays of more than 30 days were associated with nosocomial MRSA infection. Their findings are further supported by Siddiqui and Koirala (2020), who list the following additional risk factors:

- ICU admission
- Recent antibiotic use
- MRSA colonization
- Invasive procedures
- Infection with HIV
- Nursing home admission
- Open wounds
- Haemodialysis
- Long-term indwelling catheter

Additionally, healthcare workers who come into contact with patients infected with MRSA are themselves at greater risk of infection.

Clostridium difficile

Clostridium difficile infection (CDI) was identified in 1978 as the cause of pseudomembranous colitis and has since evolved into an aggressive hospital-acquired infection (Badger *et al.*, 2012).

CDI is an HAI that causes a range of symptoms, from diarrhoea to toxic megacolon and death (Hardy *et al.*, 2012), and is generally related to poor outcomes for patients (Song *et al.*, 2008). The infection is associated with increased healthcare costs as it increases average length of stay, and for every 10 patients that acquire CDI in hospital, one will die (Forster *et al.*, 2010). It is the most common cause of nosocomial antibiotic-associated diarrhoea and pseudomembranous colitis globally, and the incidence, severity, and healthcare costs are rising, making *C. difficile* a major public health threat (Chandrasekaran and Lacy,

2017). It is the use of antibiotics that disrupt the gut flora that typically supports the proliferation of CDI and thus results in infection. Traditional treatments with metronidazole and vancomycin do not eradicate the pathogen, with 30% of infected patients experiencing recurrence (Chandrasekaran and Lacy, 2017). Treatment includes the prudent prescription of antibiotics, early isolation of patients, good hand hygiene, the use of personal protective equipment, and deep cleaning of the environment. As antibiotics are seen to be part of the problem and may predispose a patient to CDI, it is important to implement guidelines for the appropriate use of antibiotics, and broad-spectrum antibiotics should be avoided.

COVID-19 and HAIs

In one of a number of recent research articles, Rickman *et al.* (2020) report the definite or probable hospital-acquired infection of patients with COVID-19 in a major London teaching hospital. The cases were identified between 2 March 2020 and 12 April 2020, with 66 of 435 (15%) of infections thought attributable to hospital-acquired infection. As these figures were identified early on in the pandemic, the numbers will likely have continued to rise.

Figures from the Office for National Statistics (ONS, 2021) show that 883 health and social care workers died between March and December 2020. As the data only covers the period between March and December 2020, and only accounts for people aged 20–64 years in England and Wales, the true number of deaths across healthcare workers in the UK is likely to be significantly higher.

Lost on the Frontline, an online project between Kaiser Health News and *The Guardian* newspaper, identified 3,373 deaths from COVID-19 in healthcare workers in the United States as of 3 February 2021.

The physical and mental impact on healthcare workers worldwide is staggering and the long-term costs are yet to be counted.

Psychological impact of acquiring an HAI

In the first meta-analysis to estimate the impact of isolation on patient psychological wellbeing using validated depression and anxiety scales, Sharma *et al.* (2020) purport that isolation may be associated with higher rates of anxiety, depression, and several negative psychological measures. Furthermore, they estimated the per day cost of anxiety and depression in terms of quality-adjusted life years (QALYs) to be US$9.83.

Activity 2.3

- Have you worked in a healthcare facility where either MRSA or CDI was diagnosed?
- How many patients were infected?
- How did your organization deal with the infection?
- Was this appropriate?

Ventilator-associated pneumonia

Ventilator-associated pneumonia (VAP) is a common hazardous complication in mechanically ventilated patients and is associated with increased morbidity and mortality in critically ill patients (Sinuff et al., 2013). VAP is defined as pneumonia that occurs in mechanically ventilated patients more than 48–72 hours after endotracheal intubation (Gu et al., 2012). Early-onset VAP occurs 48–96 hours after intubation, and late-onset VAP is usually seen 96 hours after intubation (Augustyn, 2007).

VAP is the most common infection seen in ICUs and accounts for a quarter of all infections in critically ill patients and half the antibiotic prescriptions in mechanically ventilated patients. In addition to being a financial burden in ICUs due to increased length of stay and associated costs, it continues to contribute significantly to the morbidity and mortality of ICU patients, with an estimated attributable mortality rate of 8%–15% (Ashraf and Ostrosky-Zeichner, 2012). This figure has only dropped slightly in the past eight years, with Papazian, Klompas, and Luyt (2020) suggesting a figure of 10%, with higher mortality rates in surgical ICU patients.

COVID-19 and VAP

COVID-19 has accounted for a serious increase in VAP. Llitjos et al. (2021) undertook a retrospective multicentre cohort study of all patients admitted to seven ICUs with severe COVID-19 during the first surge in France. The aim of their research was to determine whether patients with severe COVID-19 were at higher risk of developing ICU-acquired pneumonia. They found that COVID-19 seemed to be an independent risk factor of ICU-acquired pneumonia in ventilated patients.

In their editorial published in April 2020, Cox et al. (2020) state that patients with COVID-19 are kept on ventilators for long periods of time, thus increasing their chances of acquiring nosocomial and ventilator-associated infection. This is supported by François et al. (2020) in their editorial published on 5 June 2020. They state that patients with COVID-19 often need prolonged mechanical ventilation in a prone position with heavy sedation. As a result, there is a high risk of secondary nosocomial infections, in particular ventilator-associated pneumonia. Due to the presence of "multiple clinical entities" (François et al., 2020: 1), there was, at 6 June 2020, no agreement on diagnostic strategies for VAP. Dudoignon et al. (2020), in their study of 54 patients admitted to a surgical ICU in Paris, France and published 10 days later (that is, 16 June 2020), further reported a significant rate of bacterial pneumonia, mostly late-onset VAP, in COVID-19 patients having been ventilated for more than five days.

Violence, bullying, and aggression

Healthcare workers encounter physical assaults and non-physical violence across the globe. Workplace aggression is defined as "an individual's or individuals' behaviour within or outside an organisation that is intended to physically or psychologically harm a worker or workers and occurs in a work-related setting" (Schat and Kelloway, 2005: 191). The Health and Safety Executive (HSE) defines workplace violence as: "Any incident in which a person is abused, threatened or assaulted in circumstances relating to their work" (HSE, 2020). Workplace violence may be physical or psychological, the latter referring to verbal abuse, bullying, and sexual or racial harassment (Schat and Kelloway, 2005). Workplace violence has a negative impact, with healthcare workers suffering from poor quality of life, reduced job satisfaction, stress, anxiety, burnout, accidents, and even death (Nowrouzi-Kia, 2017). According to Jiao *et al.* (2015), the main offenders are patients, their families, and visitors, dissatisfied with lines of communication, poor treatment, the attitude of healthcare workers, and long waiting times.

Liu *et al.* (2019) carried out a systematic review and meta-analysis of 254 eligible studies with a total of 331,554 participants. They found that 61.9% of participants reported exposure to some form of workplace violence, 42.5% reported exposure to non-physical violence, and 24.4% reported experiencing physical violence in the past year. Verbal abuse (57.6%) was the most common form of non-physical violence, followed by threats (33.2%) and sexual harassment (12.4%), Reports of violence differed greatly between countries, practice settings, and occupations. Liu *et al.* found the incidence of workforce violence to be especially high in Asian and North American countries, in psychiatric and emergency department settings, and among nurses and physicians. They concluded that there is a need for governments, policy-makers, and health institutions to take actions to address workplace violence towards healthcare professionals globally.

Because workplace violence is a major concern in China, Lu *et al.* (2020) undertook a meta-analysis of 47 studies covering 81,771 healthcare workers. The prevalence of violence reported was as follows:

* Physical violence   13.7%
* Psychological violence   50.8%
* Verbal abuse   61.2%
* Threats   39.5%
* Sexual harassment   6.3%

Males were more likely to be the victims of physical violence than women (23.2% vs. 12.2%); the same was true of sexual harassment (9.6% vs. 6.5%). Furthermore, workplace violence differed across specialities:

* Emergency medicine   79.8%
* Paediatrics   73.7%
* Surgery   62.4%
* Gynaecology   61.1%

COVID-19 and violence, bullying, and aggression

Many experts argue that COVID-19 is the greatest threat to public health since the 1918 influenza outbreak and that it has challenged our daily lives, society, economic stability, and behaviours. Healthcare workers globally have been exposed to hazards that put their lives, and consequently the lives of their families, at risk on a daily basis. Apart from exposure to COVID-19, they face psychological stress, long working hours, exhaustion, and burnout. They are constantly fearful that they will transmit the virus to members of their families, and face stigmatization and ostracism when treating patients. Over and above this, it seems that they are also facing violence at work. In a study carried out in Mexico and published in May 2020, Rodríguez-Bolaños *et al.* reported that there has been an increase of violence against healthcare workers who are thought to have spread the virus. Patients have been seen to cough on and/or spit at healthcare workers. Additionally, healthcare workers in Mexico have been forced to travel to work on bicycles as they were being denied access to public transport (Bagcchi, 2020). Rodríguez-Bolaños *et al.* (2020) suggest that there is a need for further studies to understand and prevent such violence in an infectious disease context. Similarly, Elhadi *et al.* (2020) reported verbal abuse towards physicians providing care during the COVID-19 outbreak and civil war in Libya. Devi (2020) noted that the International Committee of the Red Cross (ICRC) reported in a statement dated 18 August 2020, that they had been notified of more than 600 incidents of violence against healthcare workers. The head of ICRC's Health Care in Danger initiative told *The Lancet*: "Unfortunately, these figures were not a surprise because violence is often exacerbated by emergencies. We know from cross-sectional studies that the majority of health workers have experienced violence in the workplace that varies from country to country and their thresholds of violence" (Devi, 2020: 658). However, in the UK the experience of stigma resulting in violence appears to be different, with members of the public, in the main, truly appreciating the work undertaken by healthcare workers (Bagcchi, 2020).

Activity 2.4

- Have you been the victim of violence, bullying, or aggression?
- What systems are in place in your workplace to reduce this?
- What else can be done to reduce the incidence of violence, bullying, and aggression where you work?

Pressure ulcers

Pressure ulcers are a common but usually preventable condition most often seen in older adults. The National Pressure Advisory Panel defines a pressure ulcer as "localized damage to the skin and underlying soft tissue usually over a bony prominence or related to a medical or other device … as a result of intense and/or prolonged pressure or pressure in combination with shear" (Edsberg *et al.*, 2016: 585). In adults, pressure ulcers are commonly found on bony prominences in the sacral and hip areas, although they are also found in the lower extremities in approximately 25% of cases. As many as 25% of neonatal and paediatric patients hospitalized in an ICU also suffer from pressure ulcers, mainly over the occipital bone (Baharestami and Ratliff, 2007). Hospital-acquired pressure ulcers have a major impact on the health status of infants and children (Murray *et al.*, 2013)

Mervis and Phillips (2019) state that the incidence of pressure ulcers has not been reduced significantly over the past 20 years and that they affect 1–3 million adults per annum in the USA, resulting in reduced quality of life, increased morbidity, and mortality. The cost of care has risen over this period of time. Whilst affecting patients in general hospital settings, pressure ulcers are more prevalent in ICUs. Patients with neurological impairment have a 25–85% risk of pressure ulcers.

At-risk populations include:

• Adults, children, and neonates
• Bedbound or wheelchair bound patients with impaired mobility or sensation
• Elderly patients with normal skin changes associated with ageing

COVID-19 and pressure ulcers

COVID-19 has highlighted a number of issues associated with tissue viability. Foremost among them is the stark impact of device-related pressure ulcers in healthcare workers wearing face masks for long periods of time and patients on continuous positive airway pressure (CPAP) and/or invasive ventilation (Gefen and Ousey, 2020).

For healthcare workers, typically one-size-fits-all applies, meaning that the stiff material of FFP3 masks makes them uncomfortable to wear and PPE-related pressure ulcers introduce the risk of bacterial, fungal, and viral (including COVID-19) infection, with possible fatal results (Gefen, 2020). Damage to the nasal bridge, cheeks, and forehead is most prevalent in those wearing masks and visors.

For patients suffering from COVID-19, the ICU inpatient stay is relatively long. Diagnosis and treatment of COVID-19 patients will require one or more of the following medical devices, all of which are strongly associated with device-related pressure ulcers (Gefen and Ousey, 2020):

• Continuous positive airway pressure (CPAP) masks
• Endotracheal tubes and fixators
• Nasogastric tubes
• Oxygen saturation probes
• Temperature probes
• ECG electrodes

- Arterial lines
- Other intravenous cannulas
- Blood pressure cuffs
- Urinary catheters
- Faecal containment devices
- Identity bands

In severe cases of acute respiratory distress syndrome (ARDS), as in COVID-19, invasive ventilation in the prone position improves the prognosis but also increases the risk of facial ulcers. In the case of a 50-year-old woman discussed by Zingarelli *et al.* (2020), it was noted that after 15 days in ICU, she was suffering from multiple facial skin lesions and necrosis involving her lips, chin, perioral area, both cheeks, left zygomatic region, and superior and inferior left eyelids. A plastic surgery evaluation was requested and recommendations made, but one week later her condition worsened, a tracheostomy was performed, and her skin lesions improved.

Psychological impact of pressure ulcers

Some researchers have shown an interest in the psychological impact of pressure ulcers. Gorecki *et al.* (2012) conducted a systematic review in which they reviewed the responses of 2,463 adults with pressure ulcers in hospitals, the community, and long-term care settings. Their research spanned Europe, the Unites States, Asia, and Australia. They found that pressure ulcers had a significant impact on patients and their families and quality of life. The research also highlighted what patients see as social isolation, as they are concerned about what others will think about wound leakage and smell.

Patients with pressure ulcers tend to have a longer length of stay than patients without such ulcers. Pain, a decrease in independence, and anxiety have all been reported as common (Gorecki *et al.*, 2012).

Activity 2.5

- Have you treated a patient with a pressure ulcer?
- Access the articles by Boesch *et al.* (2012) and Visscher *et al.* (2013) to see how you might lead a quality improvement project to reduce the incidence of pressure ulcers in your workplace.

Medication errors

Whilst many medication errors cause little or no harm, some can cause great harm, and all are preventable (Agrawal *et al.*, 2009). Medication errors occur in all settings and at all levels of care.

Elliott *et al.* (2021) estimate that 237 million medication errors occur annually in England in primary care, secondary care, and care home settings. Adverse drug events (ADEs) are avoidable; 72% cause little or no harm but 66 million are clinically significant, with 34% of potentially clinically significant errors occurring in primary care. ADEs cost the NHS an estimated £98,462,582 annually, add 1881,626 bed days, and are a direct cause of, or contribute to, 1,708 fatalities. Primary care ADEs leading to hospital admission cost the NHS £83.7 million and led to 627 deaths, while secondary care ADEs resulted in longer hospital stays that cost the NHS £14.8 million and caused or contributed to 1,081 deaths (Elliott *et al.*, 2021)

Tariq *et al.* (2020) found that 7000 to 9000 deaths in the USA are due to medication errors, with many people often not reporting adverse reactions. With over 7 million patients affected and at a cost of $40 billion annually, patients experience physical and psychological pain after an ADE. Tariq *et al.* suggested the following common medication errors:

- Prescribing
- Omission
- Wrong time
- Unauthorized drug
- Improper dose
- Wrong dose prescription/wrong dose preparation
- Administration errors, including the incorrect route of administration, giving the drug to the wrong patient, extra dose or wrong rate
- Monitoring errors, such as failing to take into account patient liver and renal function, failing to document allergy or potential for drug interaction
- Compliance errors, such as not following protocol or rules established for dispensing and prescribing medications

And the following common system failures:

- Inaccurate order transcription
- Drug knowledge dissemination
- Failing to obtain allergy history
- Incomplete order checking
- Mistakes in the tracking of medication orders
- Poor professional communication
- Unavailable or inaccurate patient information

In the first systematic review of the epidemiology of medication errors and medication-associated errors in community settings, Assiri *et al.* (2018) investigated medication errors in adults in primary care, ambulatory care, and in their homes. Searching six international databases (CINAHL, EMBASE, Eastern Mediterranean Regional Office of the WHO, MEDLINE, PsycINFO, and Web of

Science – together with Google Scholar) for articles published between 1 January 2006 and 31 December 2015, 60 studies met their inclusion criteria: 53 focused on medication errors, 3 on error-related adverse effects, and 4 on risk factors only. Included studies were conducted in the following regions:

- Asia   9 studies
- Australia   4 studies
- Europe   32 studies
- North America   8 studies
- South America   5 studies
- Across continents   2 studies

And in the following settings:

- Primary healthcare   19
- Community or home   14
- Ambulatory care or outpatients 16
- Community pharmacies   5
- Post discharge settings   2

These authors' findings showed a very wide range (2–94%) of medication errors, probably due to inconsistences in the definition of medication errors, populations studies, and differing outcome measures. The most common patient-related risk factors were the number of medications prescribed and the advancing age of patients.

Ying, Qian, and Kun (2020) reported that as of 3 April 2020, no medication errors had occurred in Jilin Province in Northeast China during the COVID-19 pandemic.

Falls in the elderly

People are living longer and falls are a leading cause of injury and death in the elderly (Huang *et al.*, 2012); thus falls are considered a major public health issue in older people (Palvanen *et al.*, 2013). This statement is further supported by Alshamarri *et al.* (2018), who write that falls in the elderly within healthcare organizations are one of the major causes of injury and deaths globally and, after road traffic accidents, are the second main cause of unintentional deaths.

This group of patients fall for a number of reasons, including:

- Changes in physical function, for example vision and hearing, and physiology
- Changes to balance and gait
- The use (and misuse) of medications to manage polymorbidity

Falls in the elderly living in the community

Pavlovic *et al.* (2017) compared falls in the elderly in the community with falls in the elderly living in institutions. They conducted their study between 1 May 2015 and 1 December 2015 and included 300 community-dwelling elderly patients and 110 nursing home residents. They found that the incidence of falls was higher in nursing homes. They noted a number of risk factors, including malnutrition among community-dwelling elderly who also suffered from urinary incontinence more frequently. Assistance in basic activities of daily living was required by 8.3% of community-dwelling elderly and 3.9% of nursing home residents. Risk factors in both groups included visual and hearing difficulties, urinary incontinence, damaged functional status, malnutrition, and the use of more than three medications per day. Despite community-dwelling elderly seeming to be more at risk of falls, the converse was true.

Falls in hospitalized elderly

Cartagena *et al.* (2017), stating that the literature related to inpatient mortality of falls in the elderly is limited, undertook a study to examine associated risk factors. They examined the case records of patients admitted to a regional trauma centre in the United States between 2003 and 2013. In total, 1,026 elderly patients aged 80.94 ± 8.16 years (mean ± standard deviation) were admitted, 77% of whom had at least one comorbidity. The bulk of the falls occurred at home and more than half of the patients fell from ground level. The inpatient mortality rate was 16%, with head injury being the most common injury in patients who died (77%). In addition to age, the Injury Severity Score (ISS), Glasgow Coma Scale (GCS) score, ICU admission, and anaemia were all significantly related to morbidity in this group of patients. Cartagena *et al.* concluded that ground level falls in the elderly are associated with a significant mortality rate. In addition, elderly patients with anaemia were twice as likely to die in hospital after a fall.

Psychological impact falls in the elderly

Mézière *et al.* (2020) reported that falls in the elderly result in serious psychological issues, with reduced quality of life, fear of falling, and low self-esteem.

Suicide

In-patient suicide

Whilst not reported in the NHS Never Events report (2020), inpatient suicide appears to be an issue in both Hong Kong and the United States.

The Hong Kong Hospital Authority (2020) reported six cases of suicide between October 2019 and September 2020:

- A lymphoma patient with progressive disease and with previous mental health illness and suicidal ideations. Eight days after admission and two days prior to discharge, the patient jumped from a height
- A patient with adenocarcinoma of the lung and extensive metastases was found hanging two days after admission
- A patient with recently diagnosed colorectal cancer and metastases and a history of depression, although not considered a suicide risk at the time of admission, left the ward to go shopping. When the patient did not return, the police were informed and the patient was found hanging at home
- A patient with Stage III olfactory neuroblastoma, and not considered a suicide risk at the time of admission, was found in the shower cubicle with the shower hose around the neck
- A patient with sigmoid colon cancer, having declined chemotherapy at the time of surgery in 2018, was referred to hospice care. On day 15 after admission, and during the night, the patient suffocated using a vomit bag
- A patient with persistent cough, not considered a suicide risk at the time of admission, jumped from a height three days after admission

In the United States, Williams *et al.* (2018) reported that estimates of inpatient suicide are unreliable. In order to form a better understanding of the prevalence of suicide, they studied two data sets. Using a cross-sectional analysis of data from 27 states reporting to the National Violent Death Reporting System (NVDRS) for 2014–2015 and from hospitals reporting to The Joint Commission's Sentinel Events (SE) (2020) database from 2010 to 2017, they identified and coded suicide in inpatients.

Interrogation of the NVDRS during 2014–2015 demonstrated that 73.9% of inpatient suicides occurred during psychiatric treatment with an estimate of between 48.5 and 64.9 inpatient suicides per year. Of these, 31.0 to 51.7 involved psychiatric patients. Hanging was the most common method of suicide reported in both the NVDRS and the SE databases, at 71.7% and 70.3% respectively.

The authors conclude that these figures are significantly below the estimated numbers of suicides, which is thought to be 1,500 per annum. They recommend that hospitals should focus on alleviating the risks related to hanging together with the risk of suicide immediately following discharge.

COVID-19-related suicide amongst healthcare workers

The global impact of COVID-19 is unequalled in living memory. Health services are crumbling under the weight of illness, and this has had an unprecedented impact on the physical and mental health of those working on the frontline. Rahman and Plummer (2020) reported on six media reports in which six nurses had committed suicide. The reporting period was March to June 2020:

1 A 49-year-old nurse in Italy noted a fever and took a COVID-19 test a few days before her death. She lived alone and committed suicide before knowing the test result

2 An unnamed nurse in her twenties was found unresponsive in the ICU in a London teaching hospital

3 A 34-year-old female nurse working in an ICU in Lombardy committed suicide after receiving a positive COVID-19 test result

4 A 32-year-old male nurse, concerned about the rationing of PPE, died after an overdose

5 A young female nurse committed suicide in Mexico having been quarantined with four of her colleagues

6 A young female nurse was found hanging in her room having tested positive for COVID-19. She died in hospital three days later

Nurses are profoundly vulnerable. With insufficient PPE in many countries, they are at high risk of infection. Working long hours and under significant mental stress, there is a need for mental health support, monitoring, and advocacy.

Dutheil *et al.* (2019) note that the suicide rate amongst physicians is high, with women particularly at risk. Gulati and Kelly (2020) endorsed this claim when they reported the suicide of a New York City physician who had been caring for COVID-19 patients. The medical director of an emergency department in a Manhattan hospital, she committed suicide in April 2020 at the age of 49.

Activity 2.6

Reflect on your own area of practice:

- What are the possible quality issues in your area of practice?
- What is the incidence, morbidity, and mortality of these issues?
- How have you been involved with these issues?
- What would your role be if you were involved?

Key points summary

In this chapter, eight incidents (needle stick and sharps injuries; hospital-acquired infections; ventilator-associated pneumonia; violence, bullying, and aggression; pressure ulcers; medication errors; falls in the older population; and inpatient suicide) have been discussed, demonstrating their incidence, morbidity, mortality, and psychological impact. The fact that these issues still arise in a climate of clinical governance illustrates that we are not yet fully mindful of, and responsible for, the tenets of clinical governance. Staff need to be vigilant of the following:

- All staff regardless of grade should follow standard precautions and report all NSSIs
- Staff need to be mindful of the risks of acquiring incurable diseases through NSSIs, for example hepatitis B, hepatitis C, and HIV

- Acquiring these diseases can impact significantly on staff and their families
- HAIs, for example MRSA and *Clostridium difficile*, are potentially lethal and can have a significant financial impact on the organization. Add to this the impact of COVID-19, and what, prior to 2020, was a problem has since become a catastrophe
- VAP is the most common infection on ICUs, accounting for a quarter of the infections occurring in critically ill patients and has a significant financial impact on the organization (due to increased length of stay). Again, COVID-19 has exponentially increased the number of patients requiring invasive mechanical ventilation and therefore the number of patients suffering from VAP
- Staff working in emergency departments, geriatric and psychiatric facilities are most at risk of violence, bullying, and aggression, and their incidence is under-reported
- Pressure ulcers can occur in all patients and are usually preventable. However, a lack of resources (e.g. insufficient staff and lack of specialist equipment) and poor guidelines contribute to this largely avoidable condition. Pressure ulcers associated with mask-wearing in healthcare workers together with pressure ulcers due to the use of medical devices in COVID-19 patients have added to the distress associated with skin lesions
- Whilst many medication errors cause little or no harm, a minority can cause great harm and all are preventable
- Falls are a leading cause of injury and death in the older population in all healthcare settings. This will become an increasing problem as demographics change
- The incidence of inpatient suicide demonstrates the need for appropriate risk assessments, whilst suicides in healthcare workers associated with COVID-19 demonstrate the need for immediate, robust, and sympathetic mental health services

Implications for practice

- It is important to make sure you are cognisant of all policies relating to all these incidents
- Always report near misses and actual events and attend Occupational Health as necessary
- Be mindful of not only the physical impact but also the psychological and financial repercussions of these issues

End-of-chapter questions

1 Does your place of work have clear policies pertaining to all of these issues? Do you know where to find them? Are they written in a language that is useful and meaningful to you?

2 Which aspects of the clinical governance framework can best be applied to assist with a reduction of incidence?

See the Appendix on page 253 for suggested answers to these questions.

References

Agrawal, A., Aronson, J.K., Britten, N., Ferner, R.E., de Smet, P.A., Fialová, D. *et al.* (2009) Medication errors: Problems and recommendations from a consensus meeting, *British Journal of Clinical Pharmacology*, 67 (6): 592–598.

Alshammari, S.A., Alhassan, A.M., Aldawsari, M.A., Bazuhair, F.O., Alotaibi, F., Aldakhil, A.A. *et al.* (2018) Falls among elderly and its relation with their health problems and surrounding environmental factors in Riyadh, *Journal of Family and Community Medicine*, 25 (1): 29–34.

Ashraf, M. and Ostrosky-Zeichner, L. (2012) Ventilator-associated pneumonia: A review, *Hospital Practice*, 40 (1): 93–105.

Assiri, G.A., Shebl, N.A., Mahmoud, M.A., Alouda, N., Grant, E., Aljadhey, H. *et al.* (2018) What is the epidemiology of medication errors, error-related adverse events and risk factors for errors in adults managed in community care contexts? A systematic review of the international literature, *British Medical Journal Open*, 8: e019101. Available at: https://doi.org/10.1136/bmjopen-2017-019101.

Augustyn, B. (2007) Ventilator-associated pneumonia: Risk factors and prevention, *Critical Care Nurse*, 27 (4): 32–39.

Badger, V.O., Ledeboer, N.A., Graham, M.B., and Edmiston, C.E. (2012) *Clostridium difficile*: Epidemiology, pathogenesis, management and prevention of a recalcitrant healthcare-associated pathogen, *Journal of Parenteral and Enteral Nutrition*, 36 (6): 645–662.

Bagcchi, S. (2020) Stigma during the COVID-19 pandemic, *The Lancet: Infectious Diseases*, 20 (7): 782. Available at: https://doi.org/10.1016/S1473-3099(20)30498-9.

Baharestani, M.M. and Ratliff, C.R. (2007) Pressure ulcers in neonates and children: An NPUAP white paper, *Advanced Skin Wound Care*, 20 (4): 218–220.

Boesch, P.R., Myers, C., Garrett, R., Nie, A.M., Thomas, N., Chima, A. *et al.* (2012) Prevention of tracheostomy-related pressure ulcers in children, *Pediatrics*, 129 (3): 792–797.

Bouya, S., Balouchi, A., Rafiemanesh, H., Amirshahi, M., Dastres, M., Moghadam, M.P. *et al.* (2020) Global prevalence and device related causes of needle stick injuries among health care workers: A systematic review and meta-analysis, *Annals of Global Health*, 86 (1): 35. Available at: https://doi.org/10.5334/aogh.2698.

Cartagena, L., Kang, A., Munnangi, S., Jordan, A., Nweze, I., Sasthakonar, V. *et al.* (2017) Risk factors associated with in-hospital mortality in elderly patients admitted to a regional trauma center after sustaining a fall, *Aging Clinical and Experimental Research*, 29 (3): 427–433.

Chandrasekaran, R. and Lacy, D.B. (2017) The role of toxins in *Clostridium difficile* infection, *FEMS Microbiology Reviews*, 41 (6): 723–750.

Chang, L., Zhao, L., Gong, H., Wang, L., and Wang, L. (2020) Severe acute respiratory syndrome coronavirus 2 RNA detected in blood donations, *Emerging Infectious Diseases*, 26 (7): 1631–1633.

Cooke, C.E. and Stephens, J.M. (2017) Clinical, economic, and humanistic burden of needlestick injuries in healthcare workers, *Medical Devices (Auckland)*, 10: 225–235.

Cox, M.J., Loman, N., Bogaert, D., and O'Grady, J. (2020) Co-infections: Potentially lethal and unexplored in COVID-19, *The Lancet*, 1 (1): e11. Available at: https://doi.org/10.1016/S2666-5247(20)30009-4.

D'Agata, E.M., Webb, G.E., Horn, M.A., Moellering, R.C., and Ruan, S. (2009) Modeling the invasion of community-acquired methicillin-resistant *Staphylococcus aureus* into hospitals, *Clinical Infectious Diseases*, 48 (3): 274–284.

Devi, S. (2020) COVID-19 exacerbates violence against health workers, *The Lancet*, 396: 10252: 658. Available at: https://doi.org/10.1016/S0140-6736(20)31858-4.

Dudoignon, E., Caméléna, F., Denia, B., Habay, A., Coutrot, M., Ressaire, Q. *et al.* (2020) Bacterial pneumonia in COVID-19 critically ill patients: A case series, *Clinical Infectious Diseases*, 72 (5): 905–906.

Dutheil, F., Aubert, C., Pereira, B., Dambrun, M., Moustafa, F., Mermillod, M. *et al.* (2019) Suicide among physicians and health-care workers: A systematic review and meta-analysis, *PLoS One*, 14 (12): e0226361. Available at: https://doi.org/10.1371/journal.pone.0226361.

Edsberg, L.E., Black, J.M., Goldberg, M., McNichol, L., Moore, L., and Sieggreen, M. (2016) Revised National Pressure Ulcer Advisory Panel pressure injury staging system: Revised pressure injury staging system, *Journal of Wound Ostomy and Continence Nursing*, 43 (6): 585–597.

Elhadi, M., Msherghi, A., Elgzairi, M., Alhashimi, A., Bouhuwaish, A., Biala, M. *et al.* (2020) Psychological status of healthcare workers during the civil war and COVID-19 pandemic: A cross-sectional study, *Journal of Psychosomatic Research*, 137: 110221. Available at: https://doi.org/10.1016/j.jpsychores.2020.110221.

Elliott, R.A., Camacho, E., Jankovic, D., Sculpher, M., and Faria, R. (2021) Economic analysis of the prevalence and clinical and economic burden of medication error in England, *British Medical Journal of Quality and Safety*, 30 (2): 96–105.

Enright, M.C., Robinson, D.A., Randle, G., Feil, E.J., Grundmann, H., and Spratt, B.G. (2002) The evolutionary history of methicillin-resistant *Staphylococcus aureus* (MRSA), *Proceedings of the National Academy of Sciences*, 99 (11): 7687–7692.

Forster, A.J., Taljaard, M., Oake, N., Wilson, K., Roth, V., and van Walraven, C. (2010) The effect of hospital-acquired infection with *Clostridium difficile* on length of stay in hospital, *Canadian Medical Association Journal*, 184 (1): 37–42.

François, B., Laterre, P.F., Luyt, C.E., and Chastre, J. (2020) The challenge of ventilator-associated pneumonia diagnosis in COVID-19 patients, *Critical Care*, 24: 289. Available at: https://doi.org/10.1186/s13054-020-03013-2.

Gefen, A. (2020) Skin tears, medical face masks, and coronavirus, *Wound Management and Prevention*, 66 (4): 6–7.

Gefen, A. and Ousey, K. (2020) Update to device-related pressure ulcers: SECURE prevention. COVID-19, face masks and skin damage, *Journal of Wound Care*, 29 (5): 245. Available at: https://doi.org/10.12968/jowc.2020.29.5.245.

Gorecki, C., Nixon, J., Madill, A., Firth, J., and Brown, J.M. (2012) What influences the impact of pressure ulcers on health-related quality of life? A qualitative patient-focused exploration of contributory factors, *Journal of Tissue Viability*, 21 (1): 3–12.

Groneberg, D.A., Braumann, H., Rolle, S., Quarcoo, D., Klingelhofer, D., Fischer, A. *et al.* (2020) Needlestick injuries: A density-equalizing mapping and socioeconomic analysis of the global research, *International Archives of Occupational and Environmental Health*, 93: 995–1006. Available at: https://doi.org/10.1007/s00420-020-01547-0.

Gu, W.-J., Gong, Y.-Z., Lei, P., No, Y.-X., and Liu, J.-C. (2012) Impact of oral care with versus without toothbrushing on the prevention of ventilator-associated pneumonia: A systematic review and meta-analysis of randomized controlled trials, *Critical Care*, 16 (5): R190. Available at: https://doi.org/10.1186/cc11675.

Gulati, G. and Kelly, B.D. (2020) Physician suicide and the COVID-19 pandemic, *Occupational Medicine*, 70 (7): 514. Available at: https://doi.org/10.1093/occmed/kqaa104.

Hardy, K., Manzoor, S., Marriott, C., Parsons, H., Waddlington, C., Gossain, S. *et al.* (2012) Utilizing rapid multiple-locus variable-number tandem-repeat analysis typing to aid control of hospital-acquired *Clostridium difficile* infection: A multicenter study, *Journal of Clinical Microbiology*, 50 (10): 3244–3248.

Health and Safety Executive (2020) *Work-related Violence*. Available at: https://www.hse.gov.uk/violence/index.htm (accessed: 7 March 2021).

Hospital Authority Hong Kong (2020) *Annual Report on Sentinel and Serious Untoward Events: October 2018–September 2019*. Available at: https://www.ha.org.hk/haho/ho/psrm/SESUEReport201819.pdf (accessed: 7 March 2021).

Hospital Authority Hong Kong (2021) *Annual Report on Sentinel and Serious Untoward Events: October 2019–September 2020*. Available at: https://www.ha.org.hk/haho/ho/psrm/E_SESUE1920.pdf (accessed: 7 March 2021).

Huang, A.R., Mallet, L., Rochefort, C.M., Eguale, T., Buckeridge, D., and Tamblyn, R. (2012) Medication-related falls in the elderly: Causative factors and preventive strategies, *Drugs and Aging*, 29 (5): 359–376.

Hudson, L.O., Murphy, C.R., Spratt, B.G., Enright, M.C., Terpstra, L., Gombosev, A. *et al.* (2011) Differences in methicillin-resistant *Staphylococcus aureus* isolated from pediatric and adult patients from hospital in a large county in California, *Journal of Clinical Microbiology*, 50 (3): 573–579.

Jiao, M., Ning, N., Li, Y., Gao, L., Cui, Y., Sun, H. *et al.* (2015) Workplace violence against nurses in Chinese hospitals: A cross-sectional survey, *BMJ Open*, 5: e006719. Available at: https://doi.org/10.1136/bmjopen-2014-006719 (accessed: 7 March 2021).

King, K.C. and Strony, R. (2019) Needlestick, in *StatPearls*. Treasure Island, FL: StatPearls Publishing. Available at: https://www.ncbi.nlm.nih.gov/books/NBK493147/ (accessed: 25 June 2021).

Kourtis, A.P., Hatfield, K., Baggs, J., Mu, Y., See, I., Epson, E. *et al.* (2019) Vital signs: Epidemiology and recent trends in methicillin-resistant and in methicillin-susceptible *Staphylococcus aureus* bloodstream infections – United States, *Morbidity and Mortality Weekly Report*, 68 (9): 214–219. Available at: https://www.cdc.gov/mmwr/volumes/68/wr/mm6809e1.htm?s_cid=mm6809e1_w (accessed: 25 June 2021).

Krein, S.L., Kowalski, C.P., Hofer, T.P. and Saint, S. (2011) Preventing hospital acquired infections: A national survey of practices reported by U.S. hospitals in 2005 and 2009, *Journal of General Internal Medicine*, 22: 773–779.

Liu, J., Gan, Y., Jiang, H., Li, L., Dwyer, R., Lu, K. *et al.* (2019) Prevalence of workplace violence against healthcare workers: A systematic review and meta-analysis, *Occupational and Environmental Medicine*, 76 (12): 927–937.

Llitjos, J.F., Bredin, S., Lascarrou, J.B., Soumagne, T., Cojocaru, M., Leclerc, M. *et al.* (2021) Increased susceptibility to intensive care unit-acquired pneumonia in severe COVID-19 patients: A multicentre retrospective cohort study, *Annals of Intensive Care*, 11: 20. Available at: https://doi.org/10.1186/s13613-021-00812-w.

Lu, L., Dong, M., Wang, S.-B., Zhang, L., Ng, C.H., Ungvari, G.S. *et al.* (2020) Prevalence of workplace violence against health-care professionals in China: A comprehensive meta-analysis of observational surveys, *Trauma, Violence and Abuse*, 21 (3): 498–509.

Mao, P., Peng, P., Liu, Z., Xue, Z., and Yao, C. (2019) Risk factors and clinical outcomes of hospital-acquired MRSA infections in Chongqing, China, *Infection Drug Resistance*, 12: 3709–3717.

Mervis, J.S. and Phillips, T.J. (2019) Pressure ulcers: Pathophysiology, epidemiology, risk factors, and presentation, *Journal of the American Academy of Dermatology*, 81 (4): 881–890.

Mézière, A.M., Denis, A., Berchel, N., Moreau, C., and Perrot, A. (2020) Psychological impact of Wii-empowerment in hospitalized elderly patients who fall: Pilot study, *Soins. Gerontologie*, 25 (142): 34–38.

Murray, J.S., Noonan, C., Quigley, S., and Curley, M. (2013) Medical device-related hospital-acquired pressure ulcers in children: An integrative review, *Journal of Paediatric Nursing*, 28 (6): 585–595.

NHS (2020) *Never Events*. Available at: https://www.england.nhs.uk/publication/never-events/ (accessed: 7 March 2021).

NHS Improvement (2018) *Never Events Policy and Framework*. Available at: https://www.england.nhs.uk/wp-content/uploads/2020/11/Revised-Never-Events-policy-and-framework-FINAL.pdf (accessed: 7 March 2021).

Nowrouzi-Kia, B. (2017) The impact of workplace violence on health care workers' quality of life, *Developmental Medicine and Child Neurology*, 59 (7): 675. Available at: https://doi.org/10.1111/dmcn.13466.

Ochmann, U. and Wicker, S. (2020) Needlestick injuries of healthcare workers, *Medizinische Klinik, Intensivmedizin und Notfallmedizin*, 115 (1): 67–78.

Office of National Statistics (ONS) (2021) *Coronavirus (COVID-19) Related Deaths by Occupation, England and Wales: Deaths registered between 9 March and 28 December 2020*. London: ONS.

Palaven, M., Kannus, P., Piirtola, M., Miemi, S., Parkkan, S., and Jarvinen, M. (2013) Effectiveness of the Chaos Falls Clinic in preventing falls and injuries in home-dwelling older adults: A randomized controlled trial, *Injury*, 45 (1): 265–271.

Papazian, L., Klompas, M., and Luyt, C.E. (2020) Ventilator-associated pneumonia in adults: A narrative review, *Intensive Care Medicine*, 46 (5): 888–906.

Pavlovic, J., Racic, M., Kekus, D., Despotovic, M., Jokovic, S., and Hadzivukovic, N. (2017) Incidence of falls in the elderly population, *Medicinski Pregled*, 70 (9/10): 277–282.

Popovich, K.J., Hota, B., Aroutcheva, A., Kurien, L., Patel, J., Lyles-Banks, R. *et al.* (2013) Community-associated methicillin-resistant *Staphylococcus aureus* colonization burden in HIV-infected patients, *Clinical Infectious Diseases*, 56 (8): 1067–1074.

Rahman, A. and Plummer, V. (2020) COVID-19 related suicide among hospital nurses: Case study evidence from worldwide media reports, *Psychiatry Research*, 291: 113272. Available at: https://doi.org/10.1016/j.psychres.2020.113272.

Rickman, H.M., Rampling, T., Shaw, K., Martinez-Garcia, G., Hail, L., Coen, P. *et al.* (2020) Nosocomial transmission of coronavirus disease 2019: A retrospective study of 66 hospital-acquired cases in a London teaching hospital, *Clinical Infectious Diseases*, 72 (4): 690–693.

Rodríguez-Bolaños, R., Cartujano-Barrera, F., Cartujano, B., Flores, Y.N., Cupertino, A.P., and Gallegos-Carrillo, K. (2020) The urgent need to address violence against health workers during the COVID-19 pandemic, *Medical Care*, 58 (7): 663.

Schat, A.C. and Kelloway, E.K. (2005) Workplace aggression, in J. Baring, E.K. Kelloway, and M. Frone (eds.) *Handbook of Work Stress*. Thousand Oaks, CA: Sage.

Sharma, A., Pillai, D.R., Lu, M., Leal, D.J., and Hollis, K.A. (2020) Impact of isolation precautions on quality of life: A meta-analysis, *Journal of Hospital Infection*, 105 (1): 35–42.

Siddiqui, A.H. and Koirala, J. (2020) Methicillin Resistant Staphylococcus aureus, in *StatPearls*. Treasure Island, FL: StatPearls Publishing. Available at: https://www.ncbi.nlm.nih.gov/books/NBK482221/ (accessed: 7 March 2021).

Sinuff, T., Muscedere, J., Cook, D.J., Dodek, P.M., Anderson, W., Keenan, S.P. *et al.* (2013) Implementation of clinical practice guidelines for ventilator-associated pneumonia: A multicentre prospective study, *Critical Care Medicine*, 41 (1): 15–23.

Song, X., Bartlett, J.G., Speck, K.A., Naegeli, A., Carroll, K., and Perl, T.M. (2008) Rising economic impact of *Clostridium difficile*-associated disease in adult hospitalized patient population, *Infection Control and Hospital Epidemiology*, 29 (9): 823–828.

Tariq, R.A., Vashisht, R., Sinha, A., and Scherbak, Y. (2020) Medication Dispensing Errors and Prevention, in *StatPearls*. Treasure Island, FL: StatPearls Publishing. Available at: https://www.ncbi.nlm.nih.gov/books/NBK519065/ (accessed: 7 March 2021).

The Joint Commission (2020) *Sentinel Event Statistics Released for 2019*. Available at: https://www.jointcommission.org/resources/news-and-multimedia/newsletters/newsletters/joint-commission-online/april-1-2020/sentinel-event-statistics-released-for-2019/ (accessed: 7 March 2021).

Thorat, N.D., Dworniczek, E., Brennan, G., Chodaczek, G., Mouras, R., Perez, V.G. *et al.* (2021) Photo-responsive functional gold nanocapsules for inactivation of community-acquired, highly virulent, multidrug-resistant MRSA, *Journal of Material Chemistry B*, 9 (3): 846–856.

Visscher, M., King, A., Nie, A.P., Schaffer, P., Taylor, T., Pruitt, D. *et al.* (2013) A quality improvement collaborative project to reduce pressure ulcers in PICUs, *Pediatrics*, 131 (6): e1950–e1960.

Wallin, T.R., Hern, H.G., and Frazee, B.W. (2008) Community-associated methicillin-resistant *Staphylococcus aureus*, *Emergency Medicine Clinics of North America*, 26 (2): 431–455.

Wang, W., Xu, Y., Gao, R., Lu, R., Han, K., Wu, G. *et al.* (2020) Detection of SARS-CoV-2 in different types of clinical specimens, *Journal of the American Medical Association*, 323 (18): 1843–1844.

Williams, S.C., Schmaltz, S.P., Castro, G.M., and Baker, D.W. (2018) Incidence and method of suicide in hospitals in the United States, *Joint Commission Journal on Quality and Patient Safety*, 44 (11): 643–650.

World Health Organization (WHO) (2019) *Needlestick Injuries*. Available at: https://www.who.int/occupational_health/topics/needinjuries/en/ (accessed: 7 March 2021).

Ying, W., Qian, Y., and Kun, Z. (2020) Drugs supply and pharmaceutical care management practices at a designated hospital during the COVID-19 epidemic, *Research in Social and Administrative Pharmacy*, 17 (1): 1978–1983.

Zingarelli, E.M., Ghiglion, M., Pesce, M., Orejuela, I., Scarrone, S., and Panizza, R. (2020) Facial pressure ulcers in a COVID-19 50-year-old female intubated patient, *Indian Journal of Plastic Surgery*, 53 (1): 144–146.

Exploring quality failings within clinical contexts

Mary Gottwald

Learning objectives

By the end of this chapter, the reader will be better able to:

- Identify the rationale for clinical audit
- Understand how quality circles can be used within quality management
- Identify the dimensions of quality
- Identify and use tools to analyse the causes of poor quality care
- Compare and contrast a variety of analytical tools

Introduction

The previous chapters have explored why the application of clinical governance is so important in today's practice and have discussed evidence linked to specific examples that highlight the incidence of poor quality healthcare. This chapter will begin with a brief discussion on clinical audit. Chapter 8 will then discuss and apply clinical audit in more detail. This chapter will continue by exploring how quality circles can be used to help health and social care teams initiate discussions around the quality of care provided that have possibly arisen from a clinical audit. It will then explore and critique a number of tools that can be used to analyse the reasons why particular quality issues and poor standards of healthcare arise in practice. These tools will be applied to specific examples from practice.

There are a variety of tools and theories that can be used when defining quality and analysing the causes of quality issues in clinical governance. In this chapter, we have chosen to focus on the following:

- Maxwell 6
- Three organizational dimensions
- Ishikawa's fishbone
- SWOT
- PESTLE

As discussed in Chapter 1, it must be remembered that quality is a personal construct dependent on one's beliefs and values and therefore quality can be considered to link to one's perception. This presents a challenge to using any of these tools and we therefore need to be mindful of this.

Clinical audit

Clinical audit can be defined as: "A quality improvement cycle that involves measurement of the effectiveness of healthcare against agreed and proven standards for high quality and taking action to bring practice in line with these standards so as to improve the quality of care and health outcomes" (HQIP, 2015: 10).

Clinical audit can be seen as the starting point so that poor quality outcomes can be evaluated and reviewed. It is also used to identify areas where standards are not being met and therefore practice needs to be developed and improved and so audit will be used to facilitate change. Clinical audit is then required again at a later date, to evaluate whether change has taken place and the quality of care provided improved.

Some might think that clinical audit has no part to play during a pandemic, as in the past audit has tended to be focused on such issues as A&E waiting times, medication errors, hospital-acquired infections, and so on. But this appears short-sighted. If clinical governance is important in normal times, and clinical audit is a key component of clinical governance, it is even more important during a pandemic the like of which we have not experienced before. Clinical audit will provide both a snapshot of our response to the pandemic as well as a more focused understanding. Importantly, the international scale of responses will provide an abundance of audit topics and results which can be shared to build up a picture of our global response to the virus.

Furthermore, it is likely that the process of conducting clinical audit will change. Audits that have previously relied on the physical interaction of staff may well change to a process that involves minimal personal interaction (Stangoe and Milan, 2020).

As stated above, clinical audit is an integral part of clinical governance and a key component of the process. It is one of the seven pillars of clinical governance:

1 Clinical audit
2 Clinical effectiveness
3 Risk management
4 Education and training
5 Patient and public involvement
6 Staffing and staff management
7 Using information and IT

Clinical audit is used to support and evaluate continuous quality improvement programmes that are a requirement of all NHS organizations and therefore can lead to a reduction in high-profile cases such as those highlighted in Chapter 1 (NICE, 2002). Audit is not just part of UK practice but also international health and social care practice. The significance of these quality improvement

Figure 3.1 The audit cycle

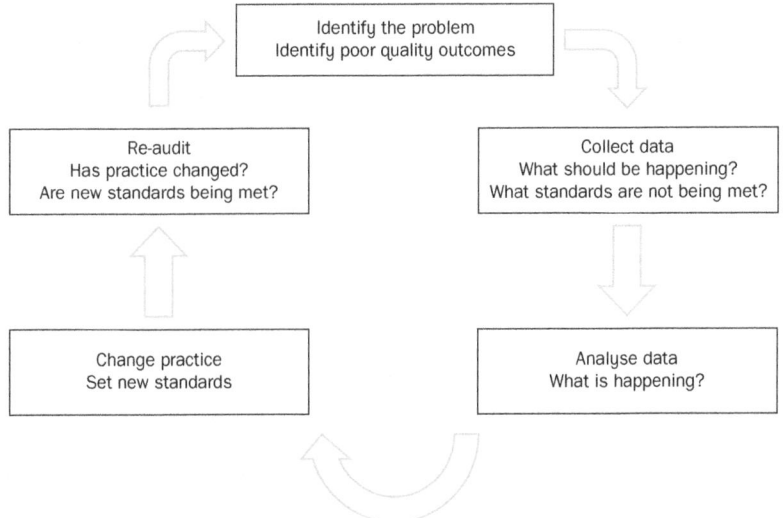

Adapted from: Benjamin (2008).

programmes is to regain public trust in healthcare services. Figure 3.1 helps to outline the audit cycle (for a more complex representation, see Figure 3.2.

The following is an example of how this audit cycle can initially be used in an orthopaedic ward in relation to pressure ulcers occurring in a patient's heels following a hip fracture:

Problem

First, using a quality circle (discussed below) the team might highlight a number of adverse events or near misses that have been reported. Following these discussions, the team can prioritize which area of practice they will focus on and improve the level of care provided, such as prevention of heel pressure ulcers following a hip fracture.

Collect data

Retrospective data will need to be collected on heel pressure ulcers following a hip fracture to provide evidence of the occurrence. This data can be used to compare with that of other organizations.

Analyse the data

The team could then use one of the tools discussed in this chapter, such as Ishikawa's fishbone, to analyse the causes. The group can discuss and identify the root causes, using the three questions suggested by The Joint Commission (2015) and listed on page 68. This will help them to decide on which of the key causes to focus on.

Change practice and set new standards

New SMART standards will need to be agreed. The following is one example of an overall SMART standard:

The incidence of heel pressure ulcers following a hip fracture will be reduced by 50% by the end of 2022.

The team might present evidence to management that supports the need for new pressure ulcer relieving mattresses to be purchased for certain patients. They might agree that further education and training needs to be organized, such as supporting staff to carry out a thorough wound assessment, supporting staff to ensure they understand how to clean wound areas thoroughly, helping staff to decide how to manage incontinence and then moisture with a skin-care regime, such as frequent cleansing and using a moisture-barrier ointment.

The team might also decide to initiate a journal club. Members can agree to read research papers and present findings to the team on interventions for heel pressure ulcers. They could decide to explore and compare interventions for heel pressure ulcers, such as a prophylactic dressing versus heel elevating devices.

Re-audit

A further audit is always required to evaluate changes to practice and a reduction in the incidence in this scenario of heel pressure ulcers. Random audit or focused audit are approaches that might be used. These audit approaches are discussed in more detail in Chapter 8.

Figure 3.2 Application of the audit cycle for pressure ulcers

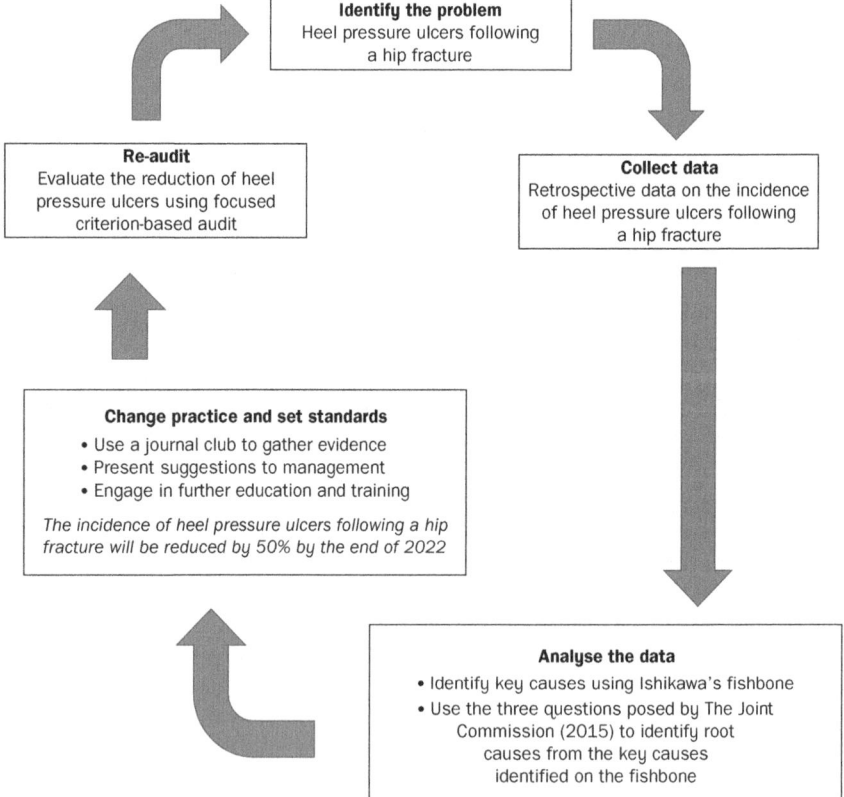

Quality circles

Quality circles were established in Japan in 1962 and in the West in the 1970s (Ishikawa, 1985). Although they originated within business, quality circles are a simple, well-used method that healthcare teams and service users can use to work together and begin discussions, for example to prioritize development of healthcare that is failing to meet required standards (such as those identified by NICE, discussed in Chapter 1). These discussions provide an opportunity for managers, service users, and healthcare professionals to share ideas, prioritize areas for improvement, and agree the way forward using clinical governance strategies.

To establish a quality circle, 3–12 volunteers, working in the same practice area, will be required. They need to have an interest in resolving specific issues within healthcare and need to agree to meet at frequent intervals to brainstorm appropriate issues (Moullin, 2002; Mullins, 2010; Sale, 2005). Ishikawa (1985) places an emphasis on the "volunteer" aspect, as this provides autonomy and empowerment for the members. He also suggests that teams should meet twice a month at a minimum, and preferably weekly initially.

There are two key members of any quality circle: a manager to help practitioners take their ideas forward; and a patient, service user, or relative, as they will have experience of the healthcare provided. Otherwise, the members can include a range of professionals at different grades.

Key point

A service user and manager are essential members of a quality circle.

Quality circles can be used both at the analysis stage and resolution stage and discussions in each of these stages will go through two phases:

1 *Divergent phase*
   - General discussion on what the quality issues are
   - Prioritization of which quality issues to focus on
   - Analysis of causes that can be used to explain why the quality issue(s) has arisen
   - Identification of all potential ways to ameliorate problem(s)
2 *Convergent phase*
   - Decision-making on which resolutions are feasible to implement
   - Decision-making on which clinical governance strategies can be used to resolve the quality issue and improve the patient experience

Divergent phase

First, all members of the group will brainstorm the various quality issues and problems that have arisen, for example medication errors, falls in the older population, pressure sores, hospital-acquired infections, workplace violence, etc. To help with this discussion, it is useful for one member of the group to agree to record all suggestions either on a laptop or flip chart. Once all the issues have been identified, members discuss the quality issue(s) that can be resolved and prioritize which will be the main focus.

It is important to remember that not all problems are necessarily within the remit of the quality circle due to resource restraints. Also, if an issue that is reasonably easy to resolve is chosen initially, then this can promote motivation and enthusiasm with the group due to a potential successful resolution (Sale, 2005).

Once the quality circle members have agreed their quality issue, the group will begin the analysis. Using one of the tools that will be discussed below, the members of the group can brainstorm all the reasons that can be used to explain the causes of a specific quality issue.

The final stage of the divergent phase is for members to identify possible strategies and resolutions, and it is at this point that all suggestions are valued and noted. The divergent phase for implementing these strategies may include some quite heated debates, because as the group brainstorm all possible resolutions, some unconventional ideas may be presented. These ideas, though, will often prompt other ideas, so can be useful.

Convergent phase

Following this brainstorming activity, the group will finally converge and identify realistic ideas that can be operationalized. An action plan will need to be identified, and it is at this point that managers can help the team by taking the ideas forward.

There are a number of advantages and disadvantages to using this method for identifying quality issues. We have highlighted the main ones in Table 3.1.

Table 3.1 Critique of quality circles

Advantages	Disadvantages
• Easy to organize	• Require planning
• Promote the consultation process	• Could be considered time-consuming
• Promote collaboration between service users and practitioners	• If not part of the formal structures, meetings may easily be cancelled due to workloads
• Teams can become involved at the local level	
• Motivate practitioners and service users	• Without the support of managers, implementing the resolutions could be problematic
• Engage multidisciplinary practitioners and service users in problem-solving activities	
• Promote understanding of different roles	• Demotivating if the recommendations are not implemented
• Provide autonomy for the members to select which problem to analyse and resolve	• Demotivating if there is resistance from senior staff
• Facilitate practitioners' understanding of quality processes	• Not part of the strategic planning level

(Continues)

Table 3.1 (Continued)

Advantages	Disadvantages
• Successful outcomes motivate and reward staff and service users. • Promote a strong organizational quality culture • Minutes are taken and therefore show positive outcomes	• Cost implications if training is required – for example, for group facilitator, group leader, minute-taker

Adapted from: Keleman (2005), Mullins (2010), Moullin (2002), and Sale (2005).

Activity 3.1

Reflect on your own area of practice:

• What would you need to do to organize a quality circle?
• How would you engage members to join the group?
• Which members would be appropriate?
• Does it matter who belongs to the quality circle?

Dimensions of quality

Two tools that demonstrate how quality can mean different things to different people are:

1 Maxwell 6
2 Ovretveit's three organizational dimensions

Maxwell argues that in order to be considered quality care, six dimensions need to be met. In contrast, the focus of Ovretveit's (1992) model is on the relationship and conflict that could occur between three dimensions.

Maxwell 6

Maxwell (1984, 1992) argues that there are six dimensions that need to be considered when contextualizing quality:

1 Efficiency and economy
2 Effectiveness
3 Access
4 Social acceptability
5 Equity
6 Relevance

These dimensions will help practitioners decide whether there is a problem with quality care or not, because if there is an issue, Maxwell considers that a quality issue has arisen. Maxwell (1992: 176) emphasizes that although these dimensions are a useful framework, they must not be taken "too literally" and are therefore perhaps a starting point for practitioners to consider. Table 3.2 briefly explains what each of Maxwell's dimensions means. Table 3.3 illustrates an example from practice where the quality of care is affected due to a failure to implement Maxwell's dimensions.

Table 3.2 Dimensions of quality

Dimension	Care is not quality if ...
Efficiency and economy	The intervention costs more than it needs to. Resources must not be misspent
Effectiveness	The evidence base has not been explored or implemented
Access	There are socio-economic or geographical problems such as access to healthcare services and difficulties getting there – can patients get the care when they need it? Are there delayed discharges, long waiting times, cancelled operations or appointments?
Social acceptability	Services provided do not meet expectations of patients, service users, and the organization. Dignity and privacy are not respected, for example having mixed wards
Equity	All those in need of the same healthcare do not receive it due to resource allocation or some form of discrimination. In the UK this could relate to the postcode lottery
Relevance	Health and social care provided is not relevant to the needs of the community

Adapted from Maxwell (1992), Barr and Dowding (2012), and Sale (2005).

Table 3.3 Worked example of Maxwell 6: pressure sores

Efficiency and economy	• Time taken to dress wounds increases the workload of staff • Complications arising due to wound infections, leading to increased time in hospital • Cost of antibiotics and infection prevention measures required following complications
Effectiveness	• Lack of assessment, for example using the Norton scale may lead to high-risk groups not being identified early • Lack of regular turning or protective barriers such as heel protectors • Failure to refer at-risk patients to the dietician for a review of nutritional levels

(Continues)

Table 3.3 (Continued)

Access	• Failure to apply protective barriers such as heel protectors correctly • Confused patients removing barriers. This may not be noticed by staff because lower limbs are covered by bed covers
Social acceptability	• Confused patients not being able to tell staff they are in pain • Patients with nerve damage not being aware of pressure areas and pain from these • Increased workloads and prioritization leading to patient voices not being heard • Lack of candour
Equity	• Regular turning not being applied • Protective equipment not being supplied • Hospital guidelines not being followed
Relevance	• Hospital processes not being adhered to • Delays in intervention

Whilst Maxwell (1992) identifies the importance of these six dimensions, a patient or service user may deem some of the dimensions to be more important than others. For example, the patient or service user may be more concerned with personal aspects such as having their operation cancelled at the last minute, or having put childcare in place following surgery so they can get to their rehabilitation when needed (access). The patient or service user may also be more worried as to whether there will be a long waiting time before their first appointment (access). In contrast, healthcare professionals may be more focused on whether the general provision is relevant to the needs of the community (relevance). Managers will have a more organizational view and therefore may be more concerned with the efficiency and economic aspects, such as whether the best treatment is being provided given the resources available. Managers may also be more concerned with effectiveness – has the evidence base of the intervention been considered?

In addition, although both the patient/service user and healthcare professional may be concerned with the outcome of an operation (effectiveness), their reasons may differ. For example, due to rheumatoid arthritis, the finger joints may need to be replaced with silicone rubber implants. The patient or service user may in the main be anxious as to whether their pain will go away and they will be able to perform activities of daily living. The surgeon, on the other hand, may be more concerned with the cosmetic outcome of the surgery.

Key point

Service users, healthcare professionals, and managers may have different values.

Ovretveit's three organizational dimensions

Ovretveit (1992) argues that different people will have different perceptions in relation to quality; in other words, the perspective of patients and service users will likely differ from that of healthcare practitioners, whose perspective might differ from that of managers. If there is conflict between the three, this will have an impact on the quality of care (see Figure 3.3).

Client quality relates to service users being provided with the service that they want. Although individuals generally are better educated today and many have access to the internet, quality care is not like shopping in a supermarket, because clients cannot necessarily choose their healthcare provision. Professional quality concerns the viewpoint that the service does meet the needs of the service user as assessed by the professionals. This is because the professionals have the knowledge and skills and understand the evidence base of practice. Management quality refers to the resources. Managers manage the budget for all resources and therefore have to use these effectively to meet the service user's needs. One of the complexities of this, though, is that resources are finite.

So, for example, an individual in the UK with multiple sclerosis may read about the effects that cannabis has on spasticity and therefore request this intervention to be provided free of charge on the NHS. However, the professionals may understand that the evidence base linked to this is weak and the managers may consider the cost too high in relation to the number of patients wanting this intervention. This illustrates that there is conflict between these three parties and so care is not considered to be of high quality from the patient's perspective.

Figure 3.3 Three organizational dimensions

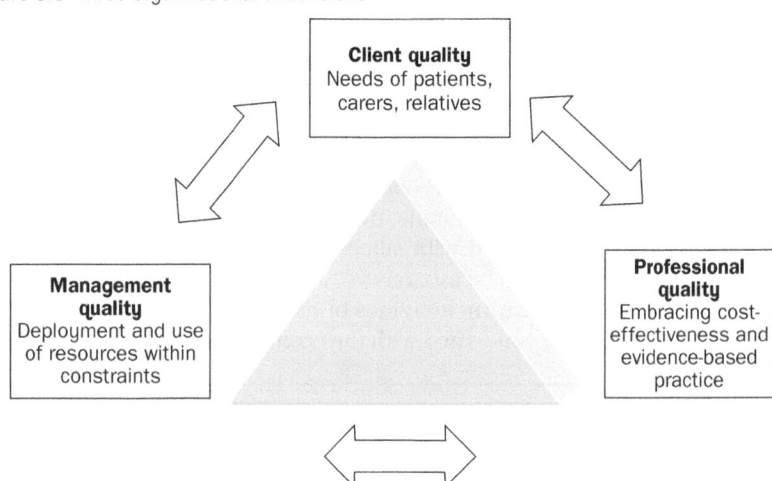

Adapted from: Ovretveit (1992).

> **Key point**
>
> Quality care must not involve conflict between the service user, professional, or management.

Another example published in the UK media in 2012 illustrates how some individuals are denied cancer medication due to the high cost of some drugs. Such a situation also demonstrates conflict between managers, professionals, and patients. The managers and professionals are likely to be focused on the resources involved in cost and efficacy of treatment, whilst the patients want what they see to be the most effective treatment. This conflict can result in patients moving home, the media becoming involved, and general patient dissatisfaction. In this example, the patient went to the press and treatment was given without his having to move to a different postcode.

A more recent international example occurred during the coronavirus pandemic in 2020. There was a global shortage of personal protective equipment (PPE). The conflict between the supply chains/wider management, professionals, and patients was clearly linked to patients and staff catching COVID-19. There was also conflict linked to the increase in cost of PPE, with the potential result that poorer countries would be unable to afford to purchase sufficient PPE, thus putting staff and patients at risk. The WHO shipped millions of items of PPE to 47+ countries, though due to time constraints and costs, supplies were quickly in danger of running out.

Having explored the dimensions of quality that need to be considered, we now discuss and apply a number of tools that could be used to analyse the causes.

Ishikawa's fishbone

Ishikawa (1985) initiated a simple method that can be used to explain the causes of quality issues through either a root cause analysis or a cause-and-effect analysis. The aim of this tool is to identify all the causes of the problem systematically, using a fish shape to explore the causes. The problem is illustrated as being in the head of the fish and each cause as being on one of the bones of the fish. This is known as a cause-and-effect analysis.

If practitioners and patients want to do a more in-depth root cause analysis, the causes of every item listed on the bones are identified separately. For example, Figure 3.4 as it stands is a cause-and-effect diagram. The same diagram can be used as a root cause analysis if all the items listed are discussed, for example the causes of poor lighting, the causes of no British National Formulary (BNF), the causes of interruptions, and so on. This becomes the root cause analysis in which the analysis becomes more complex. Groups may prefer to focus initially on using this tool as a cause-and-effect tool.

Two of the causes from each of Figures 3.4 and 3.5 have been analysed further and are presented in Figures 3.6 and 3.7. One can begin to see how carrying out a root cause analysis is more complex and time-consuming; however, this more in-depth analysis would enable staff to understand which causes to aim to ameliorate first.

Key points

- The fishbone can be used to analyse causes of quality issues
- Either a root cause analysis or cause-and-effect analysis can be completed

---

The headings used on the fishbone will depend on the problem being analysed. For example, if you were exploring the reasons behind high staff turnover in a healthcare organization, you might choose the following headings:

- Economy
- Performance of the organization
- Organizational culture
- Job characteristics
- Unrealistic employee expectations
- Personal reasons

Some often-used headings are:

- Methods, manpower, materials, machines
- Place, policies, people, procedures
- Surroundings, suppliers, systems, skills

To illustrate how the fishbone could be used, we have chosen to use the four Ps: place, policies, people, and procedures.

Worked examples of Ishikawa's fishbone: medication errors and pressure sores

Chapter 2 discussed the recent evidence that shows that medication errors and pressure sores are common international quality issues within healthcare practice. Nourian *et al.* (2020) go further and state that medication errors are the most common of all errors in healthcare and thus their research looked at why staff did not report errors. Their research was conducted in neonatal intensive care in Tehran, Iran. In total, 166 nurses with at least one year's experience took part in this cross-sectional survey and questionnaires were used to collect the data. Nine questionnaires were not included in the final analysis, as not all aspects of the questionnaire had been completed.

The reasons why medication errors are not reported included time needed to complete incident reporting forms, nurses not realizing that they had made an error, or not thinking an error to be serious enough to warrant being reported. They also felt fearful of reporting because of the impact it might have on them, or the risk of litigation from the service user or their family. For example, if a blame culture existed in the organization in which an error was made, it might be that the nurse administering a wrong medication would be blamed outright, even though the error was made initially in the pharmacy.

Although this study explored the barriers to reporting errors, results also highlighted that nurses would appreciate being given positive feedback about the successful administration of medication because they felt this would lead to fewer errors and therefore increased patient safety. This concurs with a report published by The Health Foundation (2010), where the newly appointed CEO decided to share examples of good practice within the organization's quality improvement programme (discussed further in Chapter 4).

Activity 3.2

Reflect on your own area of practice:

- Have you made a medication error or nearly made one?
- Did you use your organization's incident reporting form and report the error or near miss?
- If not, what were some of the barriers to reporting?

Figures 3.4 and 3.5 illustrate two examples from practice related to medication errors and pressure sores, and show how the fishbone could be used to explain the reasons why these quality issues may occur within practice.

Activity 3.3

Consider the quality issues of medication errors and pressure ulcers. Some of the causes have been included in the two fishbones. Reflect on your practice and identify some further causes.

Reflect on a quality issue from your practice:

- Draw a fishbone and analyse the reasons that could be used to explain why this issue arises.
- Begin with a cause-and-effect fishbone and then take some of the causes and think about the root causes.

Figures 3.6 and 3.7 include a worked example of an Ishikawa root cause analysis for two of the causes identified in Figures 3.4 and 3.5. Once the initial causes have been analysed, healthcare practitioners need to continue analysing the causes until the root cause is identified.

Figure 3.4 Worked example of Ishikawa's fishbone to medication errors

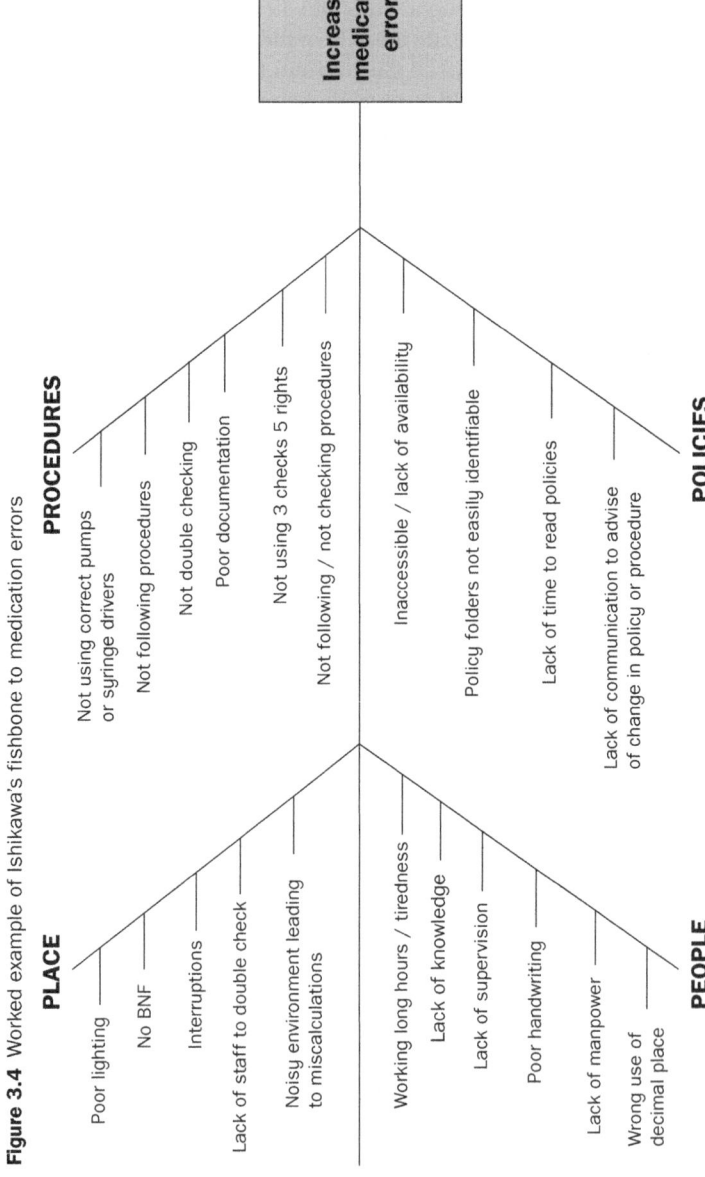

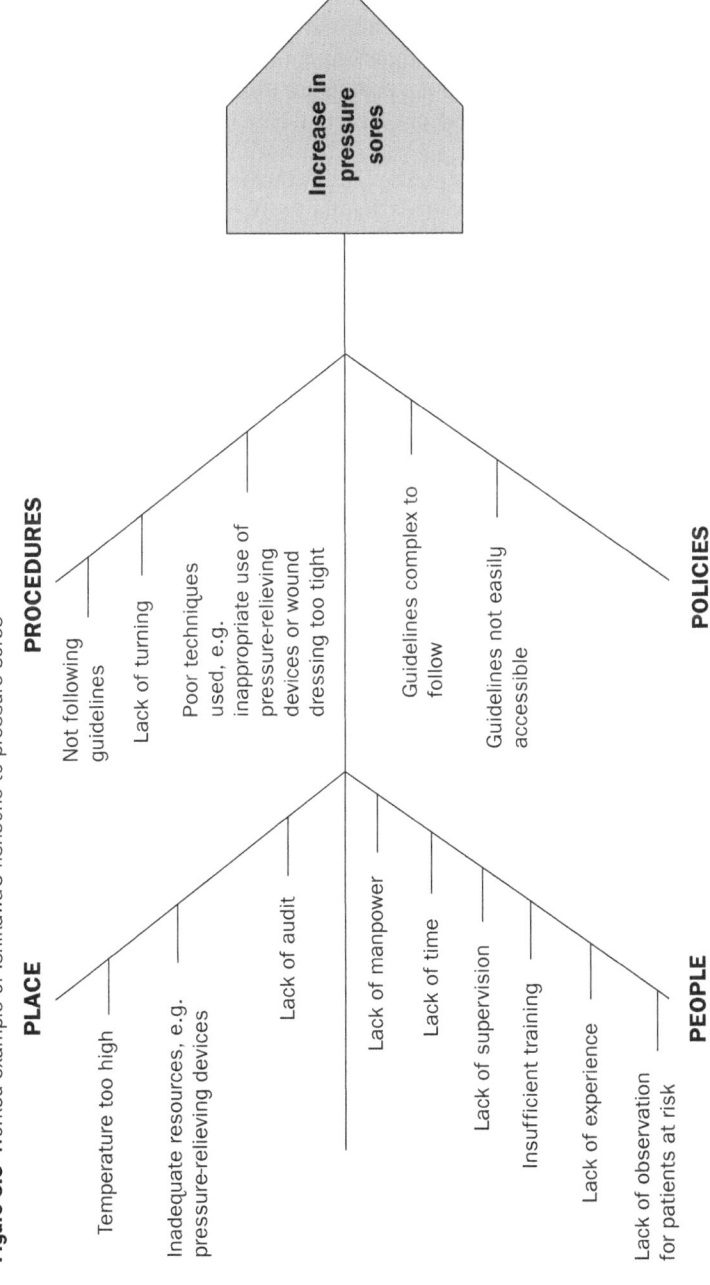

Figure 3.5 Worked example of Ishikawa's fishbone to pressure sores

Root cause analysis

It can be seen from Figures 3.6 and 3.7 that carrying out a root cause analysis can be quite complex and time-consuming. The Joint Commission (2015) identifies what might be considered a simpler way to complete a root cause analysis following a Never Event, Sentinel Event, or near miss event. They emphasize that the reason for carrying out a root cause analysis is not to apportion blame but to ensure that learning occurs, practice changes, and patient safety is safeguarded.

Carrying out this analysis can be part of the first stage of risk management – that is, risk analysis (discussed in Chapter 7). Part of risk management is about identifying how often the error occurs and the impact it has on the patient – that is, the severity of the error. So, a root cause analysis will help practitioners identify what needs to change and then whether these changes to practice are likely to lead to a reduction in the event occurring again.

The Joint Commission (2015: 7) states that there are three key questions that need to be answered in a root cause analysis:

1 What happened?
2 Why did it happen?
3 What can be done to prevent it from happening again?

The second question, why did it happen, might need to be asked a number of times in order to get to the root cause. Once these questions have been answered, it is essential for practitioners to draw up a detailed action plan. This needs to include:

• What changes are going to be implemented to reduce risk and improve patient safety?
• Who is going to be responsible for executing changes within a specified timeframe?
• How are changes in practice going to be evaluated? As with all healthcare interventions, an evaluation of these changes needs to take place (The Joint Commission, 2015)

A number of strengths of carrying out a root cause analysis have been mentioned above. However, Peerally *et al.* (2016) discuss some of the limitations of carrying out a root cause analysis. First, it is a retrospective analysis and this can be impeded by a lack of available relevant information, the passage of time, the individual's memory of the incident, or the individual's hesitancy to be seen to apportion blame. The authors discuss that one of the key considerations is who will carry out the root cause analysis – that is, should this be senior experienced personnel involved with risk management or local teams? They emphasize the need to include patients and their families in the analysis.

If the root cause analysis report is seen as the end product as opposed to the beginning, then it is unlikely that learning from the adverse event will

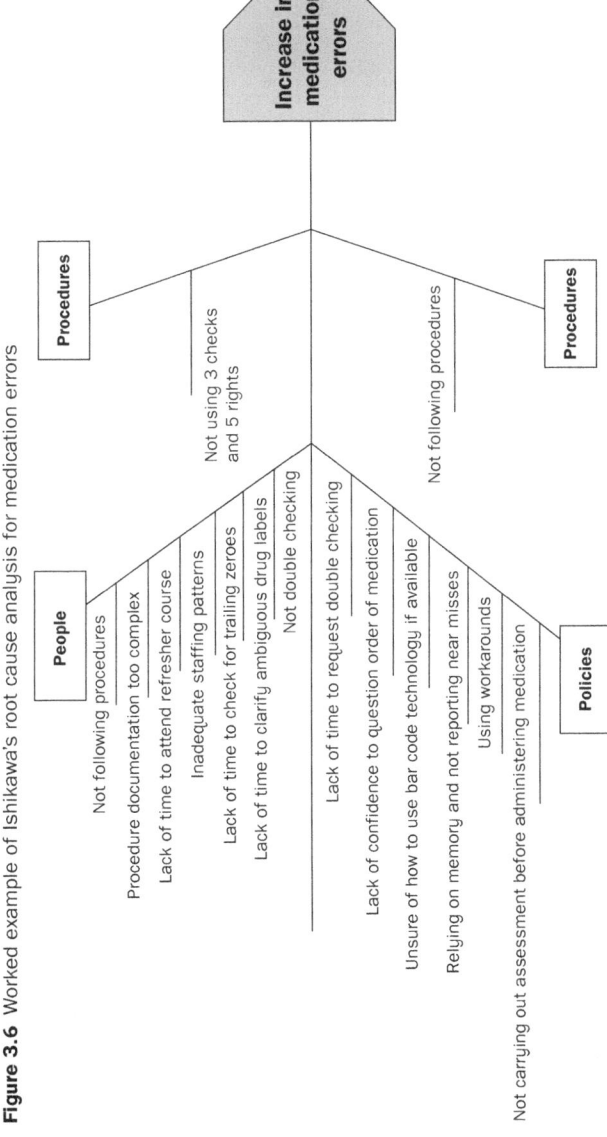

Figure 3.6 Worked example of Ishikawa's root cause analysis for medication errors

Figure 3.7 Worked example of Ishikawa's root cause analysis for pressure ulcers

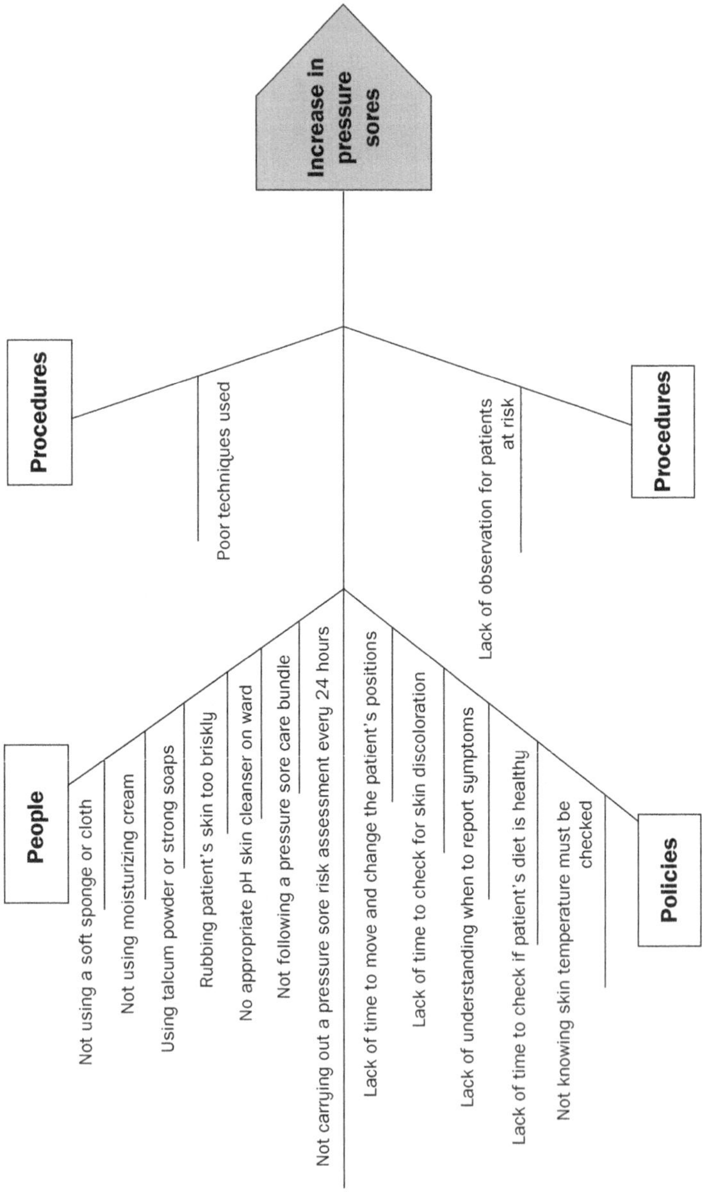

Increase in pressure sores

Procedures

Poor techniques used

Procedures

Lack of observation for patients at risk

People

Not using a soft sponge or cloth
Not using moisturizing cream
Using talcum powder or strong soaps
Rubbing patient's skin too briskly
No appropriate pH skin cleanser on ward
Not following a pressure sore care bundle
Not carrying out a pressure sore risk assessment every 24 hours
Lack of time to move and change the patient's positions
Lack of time to check for skin discoloration
Lack of understanding when to report symptoms
Lack of time to check if patient's diet is healthy
Not knowing skin temperature must be checked

Policies

follow. Root cause analysis reports will include action plans but if the action plans are not supported by senior management, frontline staff may not feel supported in implementing the plans, in part or in full. Actions agreed need to be feasible, subject to and reliant upon the available resources so that frontline staff can implement the action plan and change practice where necessary. These changes need to be formalized in best practice procedures. Lastly, outcomes from the analysis and actions taken must be rolled out and explained to those involved in implementing such plans, otherwise learning will not take place.

In carrying out a root cause analysis, Peerally *et al.* (2016) emphasize the importance of differentiating between genuine mistakes that are in need of more robust systems being in place with the aim of improving procedures, and an incident that is more worthy of blame, such as in the case of Winterbourne View (discussed in Chapter 1) – in other words, differentiating between a blame culture and a just culture.

Activity 3.4

Consider one of the previous examples analysed using Ishikawa's fishbone (medication errors or pressure ulcers) and carry out a root cause analysis using the three questions suggested by The Joint Commission (2015).

Alternatively, you might like to consider an error that has occurred within your own workplace:

- Compare and contrast a root cause analysis using Ishikawa's fishbone with the three questions identified by The Joint Commission.
- Which do you prefer and why have you made this decision?

There are a number of strengths and limitations of the fishbone and these are illustrated in Table 3.4.

Table 3.4 Strengths and limitations of Ishikawa's fishbone

Strengths	Limitations
• Visual presentation • Can be used as both a cause-and-effect and root cause analysis • Simple tool to use • Identifies causes of quality issues	• Due to simplicity of the cause-and-effect analysis, wider issues could be missed • Does not provide the solutions • Does not prioritize which problems need to be resolved first

SWOT

Another tool that could be used within the quality circle is SWOT (Strengths, Weaknesses, Opportunities, and Threats). This is a well-known tool developed by Ansoff (1987, cited in Barr and Dowding, 2012), which has been in use for over 40 years and could be used to explore the causes of quality issues. Using this tool can be an inclusive process in that staff and other stakeholders (service users, carers) can be involved in the analysis.

Chambers *et al.* (2004) highlight that the weaknesses could also be viewed as challenges, and Walshe and Smith (2011) acknowledge that some individuals may perceive strengths as weaknesses and opportunities as threats, and vice versa. Two key aspects that are generally applied when using this tool are that the S and W relate to the internal factors that impact on organizational outcomes, and the O and T relate to the external factors that could be outside the control of practitioners but nevertheless impact on the organization (Sale, 2005; Swage, 2004). However, Barr and Dowding (2012) do not make this distinction between the internal and external factors. Unlike Ishikawa's fishbone, a SWOT analysis will explore the wider aspects – that is, the strengths as well as the weaknesses, and the opportunities as well as the threats.

Key points

- SWOT can be used to identify the internal and external factors impacting on quality care
- SWOT demonstrates that not all factors are within an individual's control

---

Once the factors have been listed, each point can be discussed in relation to possible clinical governance strategies that can be used to resolve the various factors.

Activity 3.5

Thinking about a specific quality issue in your workplace:

- What are the strengths and weaknesses?
- What might be the opportunities and threats?

When undertaking a SWOT analysis and thinking about the strengths and weaknesses, Chambers *et al.* (2004) highlight a number of points for practitioners to consider, and you may have thought about the following questions in the previous activity:

- Do staff currently employed in the organization have up-to-date knowledge and skills in relation to their area of practice?
- If not, is continuing professional development accessible for all staff? Are opportunities for further learning provided and resourced?
- Do professionals understand and value the different roles within the organization?
- Is communication within the organization effective?
- Do staff have good time management and organizational skills, and problem-solving and decision-making skills?

When thinking about the opportunities and threats outside the practitioner's control, the following questions may be helpful:

- What potential career pathways could be implemented?
- What interests could be developed?
- Are there any barriers to implementing continuing professional development?
- What impact does local or national policy have on change?

In order for a SWOT analysis to be effective, it is essential for organizations and teams to identify an action plan that should detail how the strengths could be developed further, how the weaknesses could be surmounted, how the organization/team could make the most of the opportunities, and how the threats could be limited (Walshe and Smith, 2011) or turned into opportunities.

Worked examples using SWOT: falls in the older population and ventilator-associated pneumonia

As discussed in Chapter 2, falls in the older population is an internationally common occurrence and impacts on the quality of care provided. Tables 3.5 and 3.6 identify examples from practice.

Activity 3.6

Reflect on your practice:

- Use the same quality issue that you chose to examine using Ishikawa's fishbone.
- Draw a table and identify the factors in each quadrant that could be used to explain the causes of this issue.
- Does this tool provide you with more information to consider than Ishikawa's fishbone?
- What would you consider the strengths and limitations of SWOT to be?

Table 3.5 Application of SWOT – a worked example of falls in the elderly from practice

Strengths	Weaknesses
• Equipment: up-to-date hoists, chairs, footwear, bedrails, low/high beds • Experienced staff (length of service in area at least 3 years): 50% of staff • Incident reporting: staff are good at reporting falls, which helps to reduce falls • Policies readily available	• Poor falls assessment of patient on admission by nurses (looks at patient's past medical history, balance, mental capacity, medication, if there is postural drop and incontinence) • Is the falls assessment tool used adequate? Oliver and Healey (2009) state that most tools are not tested for validity and reliability • Ward too busy for adequate patient falls assessment • Lack of understanding of importance of assessment from staff due to lack of knowledge • No care plan put in place when patient is identified as at risk of falls • Shortage of staff: fewer staff per patient • Environment: slippery floors at times, poor lighting, cluttered area around bed space, patient is not always nursed in most appropriate place on ward (too far away from nurse station) • Equipment: available, but not always used • Inexperienced staff (newly qualified, little experience in the area): 50%
Opportunities	Threats
• Professional development: university modules/courses, e-learning courses (mandatory: slips and falls) • New technology: movement alarms and hip protectors available • Education and training: to highlight weaknesses	• Staff shortages due to government cuts (recently less overlap between shifts) • Limited finance for staff training • Ageing population increasing • Complex, multiple diagnoses • Policies: evidence may not be up to date • Limited resources

Table 3.6 Application of SWOT – a worked example of ventilator-associated pneumonia from practice

Strengths	Weaknesses
• VAP care bundles as a means to deliver evidence-based practice and to measure compliance • Teaching on VAPs on mandatory study days for nursing staff • Having the right equipment on the unit, such as mouth foam swabs for chlorhexidine application, electric beds to sit the patient up (30–45 degrees) • Supportive ward manager • Member of staff belonging to the Thames Valley Critical Care Network (an action group who discuss auditing of care bundles and preventative measures)	• Nursing cultures – deficiencies in clinical practice and working in certain ways that misses key points identified to reduce VAPs • Staff resistant to change to new recommended practice • Staff/patients disliking impregnated toothbrushes used in our unit • Monthly care bundle audit results demonstrating low compliance on mouth-care practice as a preventative measure for VAP • Lack of knowledge and/or education on VAPs for some staff • The VAP care bundle needs to be used in combination – all of the elements all of the time to have greater effect on the positive outcome; audits reveal that it is not • Lack of medical lead/interest to help drive the prevention of VAPs
Opportunities	**Threats**
• Department of Health's Saving Lives Programme including high-impact interventions to reduce hospital-acquired infections such as VAPs • Thames Valley Critical Care Network – quarterly meetings; representative from each unit to attend these meetings • New technologies with ventilation, different ventilation modes to improve lung compliance. Availability of extracorporeal membrane oxygenation from other units for severe pneumonias • NICE patient safety guidelines for ventilated patients	• Cost implications/limitations of resources needed to help reduce VAPs, for example endotracheal tubes with subglottic aspiration ports, continuous cuff measurement manometers • Ageing population and increased ITU admissions with comorbidities – more likely to develop VAP

Activity 3.7

SWOT is also a useful tool for individuals to use in relation to their own personal development. Thinking about your role at work, use SWOT to identify your personal strengths, weaknesses or challenges, opportunities and threats. We suggest you draw a table with four quadrants, as illustrated above. The following questions may guide you:

- Begin with the positives! What are you good at?
- What knowledge and skills would you like to develop within the next five years?
- Are there any barriers that would prevent you achieving your goals?
- What opportunities are there within your organization or external to your organization?

Once you have completed this table, you may like to discuss your findings with your line manager. Having completed the table and having discussed it with your manager, it is not the end of the process because no doubt an action plan will need to be formulated, and this will include change. Change can be challenging and the management of change will be discussed and applied in the following chapter.

Key points

- Individuals can use SWOT for personal development
- Teams can analyse causes of quality issues using SWOT

Although SWOT is a useful tool, there are a number of limitations as well as strengths to consider, some of which are identified in Table 3.7.

Table 3.7 Critique of SWOT

Strengths	Limitations
• Guides thinking	• Strategic decisions are not
• Considers the wider picture	evident from the list provided
• Results can facilitate strategic planning	• Highlighting weaknesses
• Can be linked to audit and the results can increase motivation	could be considered challenging to staff
• Can be used individually for career development or within teams to analyse problems	• Could be considered too simplistic
• Weaknesses can be addressed to improve the efficiency and economy of the organization – this links back to Maxwell 6	• Does not provide the resolutions

(Continues)

Table 3.7 (Continued)

Strengths	Limitations
• Weaknesses can be developed into strengths • Threats can be turned into opportunities • Can be used for individual development, team and organizational development	• Does not help teams to prioritize • Organizations cannot necessarily influence the threats, for example government legislation

Adapted from: Barr and Dowding (2012), Chambers *et al.* (2004), Sale (2005), Swage (2004), Swayne, Duncan, and Ginter (2010).

PEST/PESTLE

This tool explores how the Political, Economic, Social, Technical, Legal, and Environmental could be used to understand factors leading to poor quality care. Teams may prefer to use PEST if they prefer not to explore the legal and ethical factors. The example given later in this chapter illustrates PEST. PESTLE may be used to further analyse the issues highlighted by SWOT (Swage, 2004). For example, when analysing the opportunities or threats of the organization, the PESTLE acronym could be used to guide thinking regarding what political, economic, and social factors, etc., could be deemed to threaten the organization. However, this tool explores only the external factors impacting on the quality of care, unlike SWOT, which considers both the internal and external factors.

Teams could consider what local and national government initiatives hinder healthcare organizational objectives or how local patient lobby groups affect service provision. Looking at the economic factors, healthcare provision could be affected by financial constraints at either local or national level. In Chapter 1, we discussed the impact of social factors in relation to the impact that changing demographics have on service provision and the quality of care. Technological changes occur at a fast pace and if staff are not provided with the required training, this can impact on the quality of care provided. PESTLE can be used to help organizations analyse the current situation as well as helping to plan for future developments.

In Chapter 2, we discussed needle stick injuries. NSSIs are associated with a small but significant risk to a healthcare professional's career, health, and family, as well as those of patients (Pathak *et al.*, 2011). Between 1997 and 2008, a total of 3,773 bloodborne virus exposure incidents involving healthcare workers were reported to the Health Protection Agency (HPA, 2008). Table 3.8 illustrates how PEST could be used to examine the external factors.

As with all tools, there are strengths and limitations of using this one. Table 3.9 illustrates some of these.

Table 3.8 Worked example of PEST – needle stick injuries

Political	• New legislation not followed, such as Health and Safety – Sharps Instruments in Healthcare – Regulations 2013 (implemented in EU Council Directive 2010/32/EU; EASHW, 2021) • Failure to meet external standards set by NICE • Poor workforce planning leading to insufficient skill mix
Economic	• Pressure of healthcare costs leading to a lack of sharps bins • Rising cost of resources leading to a lack of manpower and therefore increased risk of needle stick injuries occurring
Social	• Higher expectations from the public • Lack of role models leading to staff taking short cuts and risks, for example re-sheathing (recapping) needles • Change in demographics leading to increased use of healthcare services
Technological	• New devices available but not necessarily purchased

Table 3.9 Critique of PEST(LE)

Strengths	Limitations
• Encourages strategic thinking • Provides a wider understanding of issues • Raises awareness of possible threats to an organization • Provides greater depth than a SWOT analysis	• External factors are dynamic and change quickly • Does not encourage critical examination of the factors • A useful PEST requires a lot of information to be collected and this is not possible in a table • The data need to be accurate and timely

---

Activity 3.8

• Compare and contrast Ishikawa's fishbone, SWOT, and PEST/PESTLE.
• Can you think of any further advantages or disadvantages?
• Do you have a preference for one of the tools and, if so, why?

It is not possible for us to discuss and apply all the theories and tools available. Readers wishing to develop their learning further could examine the following: The Pareto principle, 5 Whys Analysis, and Failure Mode and Effects Analysis (FMEA). We include a very brief explanation below of each of these and references are also included at the end of this chapter:

1 *The Pareto principle* ("80–20" rule). Applying this principle to the quality of healthcare, 80% of the errors within healthcare are caused by a few major causes (20%), so the focus needs to be on resolving the 20% of major causes because this will impact positively on the overall quality of care provided. In

2016, Naoum *et al.* concluded from their survey that a small number (20%) of service users accounted for the majority of primary healthcare consultations and hospital admissions (80%). They posited that it was therefore important for healthcare practitioners to focus on and develop improved interventions for long-term conditions to reduce pressures on primary care as well as hospital admissions. In their work, Schoenmakers and Zeiler (2017) discuss how healthcare organizations use a vast amount of energy, something of concern to environmentalists. They identified that there were a few major causes (20%) that led to unnecessary energy consumption (80%). Using a case study approach, they carried out a root cause analysis of the causes and ranked these in terms of organizational cost. As these causes were identified, an action plan was agreed to enable improvements to be made, thus reducing energy consumption.

2   *5 Whys Analysis.* This is an easy tool to use and one that is promoted by the World Health Organization. Readers might like to combine 5 Whys Analysis with the three questions that need to be answered in a root cause analysis suggested by The Joint Commission (2015) and discussed earlier in this chapter. Having identified a problem, healthcare practitioners could begin this analysis in the second stage of the audit cycle, i.e. *collect data* (discussed at the beginning of this chapter). For example, if the team identify too many medication errors, then they ask *why* this might be the case. The team can discuss and write down their ideas on the causes of the medication errors. They need to consider answers to this first *why* that are grounded in fact. Once they have an answer, they then question this first answer by asking the second *why*. This process is repeated five times and teams are likely at this stage to be able to identify the root cause of the medication errors (NHS Improvement, 2018). If the root cause is not identified, the team will need to continue asking *why*. NHS Improvement (2018) includes some useful examples to illustrate the use of the 5 Whys.

3   *Failure Mode and Effects Analysis* (FMEA). This is a tool that can be used in the first stage of risk management, that is, during a risk analysis, to analyse causes of possible quality issues such as those occurring in healthcare, thereby aiming to avert their occurrence and leading to a risk reduction in the organization.

Activity 3.9

Readers may wish to read the following to learn how FMEA was used to improve the quality of clinical trials (Lee *et al.*, 2017) and to reduce the risks linked to medication errors (Chalidyanto and Kurniasari, 2020):

Chalidyanto, D.M. and Kurniasari, W.E. (2020) Application of Failure Mode and Effects Analysis (FMEA) report of medication processing a private hospital, *EurAsian Journal of BioSciences*, 14 (2): 3257–3261.

Lee, H., Lee, H., Baik, J., Kim, H., and Kim, R. (2017) Failure mode and effects analysis drastically reduced potential risks in clinical trial conduct, *Drug, Design, Development and Therapy*, 11: 3035–3043.

Activity 3.10

When reading about the Pareto principle, the 5 Whys, or Failure Mode and Effects Analysis (FMEA), it is very important that you think critically. Consider both the strengths and limitations of these tools. For example, although Card (2016) does outline some of the strengths, he tends to focus more on the limitations of the 5 Whys tool.

* Select two of these tools and use them to analyse a quality issue from your practice: for example, hospital-acquired infections, in-patient suicide, violence towards staff, needle stick and sharps injuries.
* Compare the results of your analysis.
* Which tool do you prefer?
* What are your reasons for your choice?

Key points summary

There are a number of ways that quality issues may be analysed. These include Maxwell 6, the three organizational dimensions, Ishikawa's fishbone, SWOT, and PESTLE, each of which has its strengths and limitations. There is no prescribed tool for a particular quality issue and so a team could decide to use Ishikawa's fishbone because they prefer a visual representation of the issue. Another team, however, may choose SWOT, to encourage them to consider both external and internal factors.

* Quality circles enable healthcare teams and service users to work together to analyse quality issues. Managers, service users, and healthcare professionals meet to share ideas, prioritize areas for improvement, and agree solutions using clinical governance strategies
* According to Maxwell (1984, 1992), quality consists of six dimensions: efficiency and economy, effectiveness, access, social acceptability, equity, and relevance. If there are issues with any of these dimensions, Maxwell considers that a quality issue has arisen
* Ovretveit (1992) argues that client quality, professional quality, and management quality need to be in alignment
* Ishikawa's fishbone is used to identify the causes of a problem systematically. This can be used in its simplest form as a cause-and-effect analysis or a more detailed root cause analysis
* According to The Joint Commission (2015), three simple questions can be used to enable practitioners to carry out a root cause analysis
* SWOT encourages examination of internal and external factors impacting on quality care
* PEST/PESTLE is useful when examining the macroenvironment

Implications for practice

- Practitioners and service users need to work together to ensure that the quality of health and social care continues to improve
- Practitioners need to understand the different dimensions that could impact on quality care
- Practitioners can follow the clinical audit cycle to help them evaluate and change practice
- Practitioners need to select an appropriate tool to analyse quality issues, based on the summary above
- Whichever analysis is used, it is key that teams agree an action plan. Teams also need to identify possible clinical governance strategies that could be used to improve the quality of healthcare provision. Teams must then re-evaluate practice to ensure change takes place and an improvement in the quality of care provided can be seen

End-of-chapter questions

1 How do quality circles differ from focus groups?
2 Which would be your preferred tool?

See the Appendix on page 254 for suggested answers to these questions.

References

Ansoff, H.I. (1987) *Corporate Strategy*. London: Penguin.

Barr, J. and Dowding, L. (2012) *Leadership in Health Care*. London: Sage.

Benjamin, A. (2008) Audit: How to do it in practice, *British Medical Journal*, 336: 1241. Available at: https://doi.org/10.1136/bmj.39527.628322.AD.

Card, A. (2016) The problem with "5 Whys", *BMJ Quality and Safety Online*, 26: 671–677. Available at: https://doi.org/10.1136/bmjqs-2016-005849.

Chalidyanto, D.M. and Kurniasari, W.E. (2020) Application of Failure Mode and Effects Analysis (FMEA) report of medication processing a private hospital, *EurAsian Journal of BioSciences*, 14 (2): 3257–3261.

Chambers, R., Tavabie, A., Mohanna, K., and Wakley, G. (2004) *The Good Appraisal Toolkit for Primary Care*. Oxford: Radcliffe.

European Agency for Safety and Health at Work (2021) *Prevention from Sharp Injuries in the Hospital and Healthcare Sector*, Directive 2010/32/EU. Available at: https://osha.europa.eu/en/legislation/directives/council-directive-2010-32-eu-prevention-from-sharp-injuries-in-the-hospital-and-healthcare-sector (accessed: 7 March 2021).

Health Protection Agency (HPA) Centre for Infections, National Public Health Service for Wales, CDSC Northern Ireland, and Health Protection Scotland (2008) *Eye of the*

Needle: Surveillance of significant occupational exposure to blood borne viruses in healthcare workers. London: HPA.

Healthcare Quality Improvement Partnership (HQIP) (2015) *A Guide to Quality Improvement Methods* London: HQIP.

Ishikawa, K. (1985) *What is Total Quality Control? The Japanese Way.* Harlow: Prentice-Hall.

Keleman, M. (2005) *Managing Quality.* London: Sage.

Lee, H., Lee, H., Baik, J., Kim, H., and Kim, R. (2017) Failure mode and effects analysis drastically reduced potential risks in clinical trial conduct, *Drug, Design, Development and Therapy*, 11: 3035–3043.

Maxwell, R.J. (1984) Quality assessment in health, *British Medical Journal*, 288: 1470–1472. Available at: https://www.bmj.com/content/bmj/288/6428/1470.full.pdf (accessed: 25 June 2021).

Maxwell, R.J. (1992) Dimensions of quality revisited: From thought to action, *Quality in Healthcare*, 1 (3): 171–177.

Moullin, M. (2002) *Delivering Excellence in Health and Social Care.* Maidenhead: Open University Press.

Mullins, L. (2010) *Management and Organisational Behaviour.* Harlow: Prentice-Hall.

Naoum, V., Kyriopoulos, D., Charonis, A., Athanasakis, K., and Kyriopoulos, J. (2016) The Pareto principle ("80–20 rule") in healthcare services in Greece, *Value in Health*, 19 (7): A618. Available at: https://doi.org/10.1016/j.jval.2016.09.1563.

NHS Improvement (2018) *Quality, Service Improvement and Redesign Tools: Root cause analysis using Five Whys.* Available at: https://www.england.nhs.uk/wp-content/uploads/2021/03/qsir-five-whys.pdf.

NICE (2002) *Principles of Best Practice in Clinical Audit.* Oxford: Radcliffe Medical Press.

Nourian, M., Babaie, M., Heidary, F., and Nasiri, M. (2020) Barriers of medication administration error reporting in neonatal and neonatal intensive care units, *Journal of Patient Safety and Quality Improvement*, 8 (3): 173–181.

Oliver, D. and Healey, F. (2009) Falls risk prediction tools for hospital inpatients: Do they work?, *Nursing Times*, 105 (7): 18–21.

Ovretveit, J. (1992) *Health Service Quality.* Oxford: Blackwell Scientific.

Pathak, R., Kahlon, K.H., Ahluwalia, S.K., Sharma, S., and Bhardwaj, R. (2011) Needle stick injury and inadequate post exposure practices among healthcare workers in a tertiary care centre in rural India, *International Journal of Collaborative Research on Internal Medicine and Public Health*, 4 (5): 638–648.

Peerally, F.M., Carr, S., Waring, J., and Dizon-Woods, M. (2016) The problems with root cause analysis, *BMJ Quality and Safety*, 26: 417–422. Available at: https://doi.org/10.1136/bmjqs-2016-005511.

Sale, D. (2005) *Understanding Clinical Governance and Quality Assurance: Making it happen.* Basingstoke: Palgrave Macmillan.

Schoenmakers I. and Zeiler, W. (2017) Pareto analysis: A first step towards nZEB hospitals, *REHVA Journal*, 54 (5): 13–16.

Stangoe, D. and Milan, Z. (2020) Auditing in the age of COVID-19: Waste of resources or an opportunity we cannot afford to waste?, *Clinical Audit*, 12: 11–12.

Swage, T. (2004) *Clinical Governance in Healthcare Practice.* London: Butterworth Heinemann.

Swayne, L., Duncan, W., and Ginter, P. (2010) *Strategic Management of Healthcare Organisations.* San Francisco, CA: Jossey-Bass.

The Health Foundation (2010) *Improvement in Practice: Beth Israel Deaconess case study. How leadership and a focus on quality rescued the Beth Israel Deaconess Medical Center.* London: The Health Foundation.

The Joint Commission (2015) *Root Cause Analysis in Health Care: Tools and Techniques*, 5th edition. Available at: https://www.jcrinc.com/-/media/deprecated-unorganized/imported-assets/jcr/default-folders/items/ebrca15pdf.pdf?db=web&hash=ABB1B-44CC5F039C56AE57838AA64E349 (accessed: 25 June 2021).

Walshe, K. and Smith, J. (2011) *Healthcare Management*. Maidenhead: Open University Press.

Change management and implementing quality improvement programmes

Mary Gottwald and Gail E. Lansdown

Learning objectives

By the end of this chapter, the reader will be better able to:

- Understand the barriers to change
- Apply five models of change to workplace issues
- Understand how important leadership is in the management of change
- Understand how quality improvement programmes can facilitate change and improve patient safety

Change is not made without inconvenience, even from worse to better.
– Richard Hooker (1554–1600), British theologian
Quoted in Samuel Johnson, *Dictionary of the English Language*,
preface (1755)

Introduction

This chapter will highlight some of the challenges and obstacles impacting on change and discuss how change agents, advocacy groups, and the involvement of patients and service users can ensure the smooth transition of change. There are a plethora of change management models, and the ones this chapter will consider are: the Diffusion of Innovation model, the RAID model, the Four A's of change, Lewin's Force-Field Analysis, and Kotter's 8-Step Process model of change. The rationale for these choices is to illustrate a variety of models from the simple to the complex. For example, Lewin's model identifies the effects of forces that either drive or resist changes to practice and uses a three-stage approach from unfreezing, to change, to refreezing, whereas Kotter's model is more in depth and shows how a number of steps can be used to facilitate and change practice. Leaders are continually faced with supporting and guiding teams through changes to practice, and we suggest they might choose to use a variety of models to guide the process.

Leadership is key to the management of change and even more so throughout 2020–2021 when healthcare staff have been faced with the further challenge of the coronavirus pandemic. If nothing else, COVID-19 has led to rapid change in the delivery of healthcare and it is key that this change leads to sustainable and organization-wide improvement. To enable this, exemplary clinical leadership is required to provide a clear shared purpose, promote positive relationships, and ensure that clinical governance systems are honest, transparent, and articulated (Graham and Woodhead, 2021). It is important to remember that some systems previously accepted as good practice may require further adaptation to meet the crisis. Change is a journey, not an event (Heath and Heath, 2013) and the pandemic has required changes to practice at an unprecedented rate. It is imperative to monitor those changes to help create a new normal.

In order for health and social care practitioners to continually develop and improve the quality of care provided, there is bound to be a need for change. However, this is not a one-off occurrence because health and social care organizations continue to be faced with challenges that will likely grow and become more complex. The COVID-19 pandemic is just one example of an added challenge. Hospitals and social care organizations continue to be pressured to improve the quality of care in all areas of practice. The management of change, therefore, is an essential skill for healthcare professionals to have and this can also help to ensure that the implementation of clinical governance strategies occurs. Healthcare is changing rapidly and continuously (Carnall, 2007), with 85% of healthcare organizations undergoing transformational change every two years. Successful operation in this arena requires the successful management of change and in particular good leadership (at all levels from frontline staff to the more senior levels).

As stated above, healthcare is changing rapidly, and therefore it is essential that healthcare professionals develop their abilities to constantly adapt to organizational change (Beerel, 2009). Parkin describes change as a "phenomenon of daily organisational life" (2009: 9), so one thing that we can be sure about is that in order to improve the quality of health and social care provision, we will frequently need to be involved in change initiatives. Changing practice to improve patient care can only be seen as a positive outcome.

Changes can be linked to demographics, political and technological aspects. The demographics of populations are constantly changing with global populations living longer and thus putting pressure on uptake of in-patient beds. Also, those receiving care will often have multiple diagnoses, which can make healthcare provision complex. Due to research, treatment interventions also change and these impact on practice, which needs to be kept up to date and evidence-based. Technology also changes, with electronic patient records and the use of telemedicine just two examples. And, as discussed in Chapter 1, patient/service-user engagement, including decision-making with regards to their own care, has grown exponentially. Patients and the public now also contribute to organizational policy and planning decisions.

However, there are many barriers to change initiatives, which means that in order to avoid conflict, managers and leaders of change need to manage both the change – that is, the situation – and the staff who are affected by that change (Sullivan and Garland, 2013). No member of staff can afford to be complacent, but it is imperative that staff at all levels are supported. Only when change is embedded in the culture of the organization will change initiatives be successful.

Barriers to change

The response to change initiatives varies and ranges from complete engagement and acceptance of the change to total resistance. In this chapter, we look at the more commonly presented barriers to change, such as resistance to change, disempowerment, uncertainty, and loss. First, however, it is necessary to think about the factors that influence nurses to raise concerns about quality of care and standards of practice through whistleblowing/speaking up.

Whistleblowing/speaking up

Although some of the older literature refers to whistleblowing, the term "speaking up" is increasingly being used, as it denotes a less negative connotation such as telling tales. As stated by Attree (2007), although underreported, nurses are required by their professional body to raise concerns about quality of care. It was a whistleblower who voiced concerns that led to

Winterbourne View, a privately run hospital for people with learning disabilities, being closed because of the poor quality of care provided (discussed in Chapter 1). However, the fear of repercussions, reprisals, labelling (as a whistleblower), and blame for raising concerns prevent individuals from reporting. Reporting is seen as a high-risk/low-benefit action, and Attree (2007) concludes that, in order to promote a culture of openness, which in turn promotes quality and learning, the barriers to reporting concerns need to be removed.

Jackson *et al.* (2010) used semi-structured interviews to determine the reasons why nurses blow the whistle and their consequent experience of having done so. They identified that the participants in their study found the experience to be highly stressful, with three main themes arising:

1 Reasons for whistleblowing: "I just couldn't advocate"
2 Feeling silenced: "Nobody speaks out"
3 Climate of fear: "You are just not safe"

Although the nurses believed they were acting as required by their professional body, they felt there was a need for clarity around certain issues, such as how they were expected to act as patients' advocates, clear guidelines were required about how to raise concerns, systems needed to react more quickly and appropriately to concerns raised by nurses, and an environment of safety in which to raise concerns needed to be promoted.

The Francis Report (2013) identified that less than 70% of staff were confident about speaking up; they believed that if they did voice their concerns, it would not lead to them being addressed and or any changes implemented. It is evident that barriers to nurses and other healthcare professionals speaking up about errors continue to exist despite a key focus of provision being on patient safety. Schwappach and Gehring (2014) conducted a survey of 1,013 healthcare professionals (doctors and nurses) from eight hospitals and nine oncology departments in Switzerland, and achieved a response rate of 65%. Using hypothetical vignettes, participants were asked about the likelihood that they would speak up regarding errors and/or procedural breaches made by others. From their responses, it is evident that willingness to speak up depended on a variety of things, including the relationship the member of staff who wanted to raise concerns had with their colleagues, and the seniority of the person wishing to speak up, such that healthcare professionals in less senior positions and in non-managerial roles were much less confident about highlighting any poor quality care being delivered. Whilst Kenny, Vandekerckhove, and Fotaki (2019) identify the same barriers as those highlighted by Attree (2017) and Jackson *et al.* (2010), they also draw attention to staff feeling ignored by management, that management are trying to silence them and prevent them from voicing concerns, that there is no trust between them and management, and that they wouldn't be protected if they spoke up. Some staff even feared that they would either be demoted or would lose their job. And all of these concerns, of course, can have an impact on an individual's mental health.

Research by Levine, Carmody, and Silk (2020) in the USA supports the work of Attree (2007), Jackson *et al.* (2010), and Kenny *et al.* (2019). They also identified that the culture of an organization (discussed in the following chapter) is directly responsible for whether a member of staff chooses to speak up or not. If healthcare professionals are going to learn from mistakes that occur in practice, the organizational culture needs to encourage speaking up. Furthermore, managers need to support staff to voice concerns, otherwise staff will not report/speak up. Managers must ensure that forms that need to be completed are accessible, concise, and easy to follow, and that they respond to any concerns raised in a positive manner. It is imperative that staff are assured they will not be penalized for reporting errors. They also need to know their peers will support them if they decide to speak up, otherwise it will impact negatively on them. Also, if there is no evidence of changes being made in light of findings arising from these concerns, staff are less likely to speak up in the future.

Whilst there are clearly barriers and challenges that prevent individuals from speaking up, the advantages of doing so outweigh the disadvantages. If errors are identified and practice changed, there will be a financial benefit to the organization, including reduced costs as a result of litigation. In addition, patient safety will be improved, thus enhancing/restoring the organization's reputation, and time spent on investigations will be reduced, leading to more time available for patients and their families.

Staff need to understand that speaking up and voicing concerns is only the beginning of a long process and a culture of silence is not to be recommended. Staff may need to repeatedly voice their concerns before an investigation begins. These investigations take time and this can also lead to staff stress.

Activity 4.1

- Has it ever been necessary for you to speak up?
- Do you feel confident enough to speak up?
- If you do feel confident in doing so, list three reasons why you feel able to.
- If you do not feel able to speak up, list three reasons why you feel you can't.
- How did your colleagues respond to this action?
- How did your organization respond to this action?

Kenny *et al.* (2019) identify that there is a need for clear legislation that protects those who choose to speak up. In the UK, NHS organizations now have processes and procedures in place and there are clear support mechanisms to encourage staff to voice concerns. There are both internal and external mechanisms that practitioners can follow when choosing to speak up.

A number of initiatives have been introduced throughout the NHS. Whilst it is preferable to resolve issues internally with line managers and senior clinicians, external procedures are now in place:

- Practitioners can contact their professional bodies to seek advice
- The Care Quality Commission (CQC) has dedicated whistleblower teams who record and follow up any concerns raised with them
- The Safety Escalation Team (SET) was established in 2012 with the remit of following up concerns raised by NHS staff, social care staff, and members of the public
- NHS Trusts have Freedom to Speak Up Guardians who ensure that processes and clear procedures are in place. A national guardians office at the CQC provides learning and support to these guardians
- The *Speaking Up Charter* (CQC, 2012) and the Department of Health provide a whistleblowing helpline
- There is a Freedom to Speak Up (FTSU) legal framework and policy that supports raising concerns (Kenny *et al.*, 2019)

Activity 4.2

Whilst we recognize that readers will not necessarily work within the NHS and may well be employed in other countries, the following links are worth exploring and may stimulate ideas and discussion amongst colleagues.

– *Raising concerns*

https://www.youtube.com/watch?v=zjau1Ey0di8&feature=emb_rel_end (accessed: 7 March 2021)
https://www.nhsemployers.org/retention-and-staff-experience/raising-concerns-whistleblowing (accessed: 7 March 2021)

The first link is to a video that discusses the importance of raising concerns. The second link provides information for employers, all staff and managers, including legislation and policy.

– *Freedom to Speak Up Guardians*

https://www.hee.nhs.uk/our-work/freedom-speak-guardians (accessed: 7 March 2021)
https://www.nationalguardian.org.uk (accessed: 7 March 2021)

The first link is a short video encouraging staff to speak up and seek out the Trust guardian. The second link provides information supporting the importance of speaking up.

In conclusion, healthcare professionals must remember that they have a duty of care and it is important to speak up in order to improve patient safety and the quality of healthcare provision. "Consumer satisfaction is the measure of service quality" (Kenny *et al.*, 2019: 67), so if organizations are going to engage in continuous quality improvement programmes, it is essential that there are clear procedures for speaking up. It is vital that those wishing to voice concerns are not silenced.

Resistance to change

For some individuals, changing practice is not a challenge. They see change as an invigorating and positive experience and are therefore happy at driving any change forward (Sullivan and Garland, 2013). However, change can be a complex process and there is evidence to suggest that some healthcare professionals find managing change challenging and therefore are resistant to change initiatives (McSherry and Pearce, 2002; Sullivan and Garland, 2013).

Parkin asserts that resistance is "where change implementers perceive a difficulty in having their ideas accepted or the change is thwarted or sabotaged by others" (2009: 155). This resistance could become a barrier to the successful implementation of clinical governance strategies. Carnall questions whether "this resistance to change is really resistance to uncertainty" (2007: 3) – that is, any resistance is not due to the change *per se* but due to the individual's uncertainty about the process. For example, individuals could be concerned that they may lose their status and incur a loss of salary and therefore may become hesitant to engage in change behaviour. Lack of trust and lack of teamwork may also be causes of resistance.

In a review of 72 papers from high-impact journals and semi-structured interviews in a Delphi study, Veenstra *et al.* (2017) concluded that a number of key elements are important for successful changes to practice and implementation of clinical governance strategies. First, having a bottom-up approach is important because this makes staff feel more involved and therefore more likely to engage with clinical governance strategies. Secondly, good teamwork with different professionals sharing responsibility leads to better engagement. Thirdly, they identified the importance of having good leaders who are able to facilitate the continuing professional development of the workforce. Clear communication with all of these aspects was deemed to be essential, especially the sharing of values-based practice as discussed in Chapter 6. These aspects link nicely to the Department of Health (1998) definition of clinical governance given in Chapter 1, as they help to create an environment in which staff at all levels are enabled to provide a high-quality healthcare service, thus encouraging a shift in culture within the organization.

The results of Nilsen *et al.* (2019) concur with those of Veenstra *et al.* (2017). They undertook semi-structured interviews with 30 doctors, nurses, and assistant nurses in Sweden with the aim of identifying barriers to change and gaining an understanding of how participants responded to change initiatives. Participants either worked within a primary or tertiary healthcare setting or a hospital. Nilsen *et al.* identified that staff felt they were more likely to resist changes initiated by the management of their organization, whilst favouring bottom-up initiatives with which they foresaw fewer problems. Staff who did not feel any proposed changes were realistic or were time-consuming tended to resist change. Poor communication from management or senior staff, and a lack of involvement and engagement with planning and implementation of change also led to resistance. "Indifference to changes and passive resistance to changes" (Nilsen *et al.*, 2019: 6) were two further barriers. We have already discussed how changes to practice are continuous and time-consuming and so this is likely to result in staff indifference. Staff felt that unless a change seemed relevant to their practice, they would not devote much energy to the proposed change.

Amarantou *et al.* (2018) carried out a small-scale research project in Greece in which 200 experienced doctors and nurses working in hospitals, specifically in accident and emergency departments, were asked to complete a questionnaire. A response rate of 79% was achieved with 158 questionnaires being returned. The aim of the study was to explore three specific views (Amarantou *et al.*, 2018: 437):

1 Participants' disposition towards change
2 Participants' attitude towards change
3 Participants' anticipated impact of change

The questionnaires were designed using a conceptual framework that linked to "personality traits, job perception, job security, communication quality, participation in decision making and employee management relationship" (Amarantou *et al.*, 2018: 428).

Results showed that resistance to change might arise at the organizational level (such as the impact that power can have), team level (such as how interconnected a team is), and individual level (such as lack of confidence in being able to implement change). Two key things reduced resistance to change, namely: if participants were included in decision-making (team and organizational level) and if they felt they had the support of their managers (team and organizational level). Personality traits were also linked to an individual's attitude towards any proposed change. However, it is interesting to note that job security and quality of communication were not major concerns in explaining resistance to change, whereas they were the two factors that caused resistance to change in the research carried out by Nilsen *et al.* (2019).

When planning changes, managers and senior staff need to be mindful that resistance to change is not just linked to the individual level.

Key points

- Resistance to change is a normal part of any change initiative
- How change is communicated to staff is important
- Engaging staff in the planning and execution of change initiatives is likely to be met with less resistance
- Bottom-up approaches can reduce resistance to change
- Good leadership is essential in the management of change

Activity 4.3

Reflect for a moment upon a change that took place within your own organization.

- How did this make you feel in the beginning?
- How did you react?
- Did your feelings change over time?

Activity 4.4

- Consider why some staff in your team resist and challenge change initiatives.
- Make a list of the barriers to change.
- Have you identified barriers other than those discussed above?

You may have considered some of the following barriers to change:

- Staff may feel a change could reduce their level of power or influence and so may feel personal loss, such as loss of self-esteem. They may also feel undermined
- Staff may go through a period of uncertainty, for example they may feel that they will not be able to meet the new demands of their jobs. This is linked to loss of control, loss of predictability, and fear of the unknown
- Expectations may differ, and the benefits of change could be seen to be biased towards one group's needs at the expense of those of another. For example, if the change is seen to benefit the management structure within the organization whilst increasing the workload of staff, there is likely to be resistance to the change process
- Anything that requires the individual to readjust to their environment can cause stress and resistance. Although individuals may use denial as a defence mechanism, this should be considered a normal, healthy reaction to organizational change
- Staff may not have been included in discussions linked to change. They may therefore feel that important information has not been communicated and managers are not empathetic towards their concerns as well as their individual issues. There may be misunderstanding and distrust. For example, if the working relationship between manager and staff is tense and the manager initiates the change (top-down approach), staff may resist due to lack of trust. It is essential that the leader/manager ensures the team are up to date with what is going on

Chambers, Boath, and Rogers (2007), Kotter and Schlesinger (2008), and Sullivan and Garland (2013) identify further barriers to those identified by Veenstra *et al.* (2017) and Nilsen *et al.* (2019), such as a lack of trust, a lack of understanding of the need for a particular change and therefore a lack of consensus, a lack of resources and a lack of evidence for the need for change, or the simple dislike of the person initiating and managing the change. Kotter and Schlesinger (2008) also suggest that leaders and managers often do not take the time to explore and understand the reasons why staff resist any change.

Key points

- Leaders of change must consider the barriers
- Staff need to be supported through the change process

Managing resistance

Kotter and Schlesinger (2008) suggest the four key methods below could be used to manage resistance.

Education and communication

One of the barriers considered earlier was lack of communication and involvement in discussions surrounding change initiatives. Leaders and managers of change (change agents) could help staff understand the rationale for change through team discussions, one-to-one discussions, staff development workshops or presentations. Having a clear action plan also ensures that staff understand the timeframes and pace of change.

Participation and involvement

Change agents could take a more participative approach and involve teams in devising the change initiative and drawing up the action plan suggested above. By involving teams in the decision-making process, there is more likely to be a feeling of ownership. However, this participative approach could be seen to be more time-consuming and not realistic if the change initiative needs to be implemented quickly.

Facilitation and support

Providing education and training has already been mentioned above. Adapting to change involves emotional responses, and so a key attribute for the change agents is to have good listening skills. Human Resources may need to provide counsellors to talk with staff who may be feeling overwhelmed or having difficulties adjusting to change.

Negotiation and agreement

This is a particularly important aspect when the change initiative impacts on an individual's role, because any impact on role identity will result in defensiveness and this would be a barrier to any change initiative. Therefore, this links back to the previous discussion on the importance of communication.

Transition period for change

Change takes time and therefore change agents not only have to recognize potential resistance but also that teams will be going through a transition period, during which a number of changes to self-esteem may be taking place. Hence it is imperative to acknowledge this and to support colleagues during any change initiative, since at any one time team members could be in a different stage of transition (Figure 4.1). Barr and Dowding (2012) liken change to Kubler-Ross's (1969) five-stage grieving process (denial, anger, bargaining, depression, and acceptance).

Activity 4.5

Click on the following link to read more about the five stages of the grieving process:

http://www.businessballs.com/elisabeth_kubler_ross_five_stages_of_grief. htm (accessed: 7 March 2021)

Look back at the notes you made when reflecting upon a change that took place within your own organization. Were some of your feelings similar to these five stages?

Changes in self-esteem during periods of transition

Figure 4.1 illustrates seven stages that individuals may go through when faced with the challenges of change. No timeframe is associated with each stage, and so when working with your colleagues it is important to consider that some staff may take longer to move through the stages and therefore may need more support, whilst others will progress more quickly. For some, change can be an exciting and motivating experience; for others, change will cause anxiety.

Key points

- Staff need to be aware that others may be struggling during periods of transition
- Staff need to support each other during periods of transition

Figure 4.1 Stages of transition

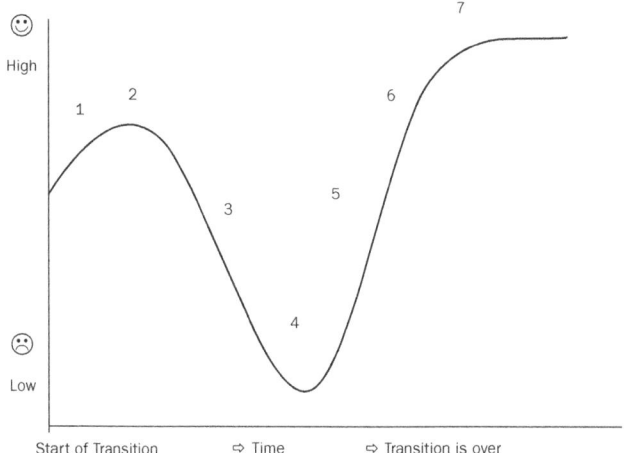

Adapted from: Hopson *et al.* (2000).

1 *Numbness*: Staff may not understand the reason behind the change and may feel shocked and unable to reason and make plans. Those who feel positive about the need for change will find this stage less intense

2 *Denial/minimization*: Changes needed may be minimized and staff may feel that the changes required are not as bad as expected. However, this could be due to the use of defence mechanisms

3 *Self-doubt*: The realities of change are now more evident and as staff become more aware, they may feel uncertainty and self-doubt. However, for some, this stage is also associated with high energy

4 *Acceptance of reality/letting go*: Moving through the first three stages will have involved some attachment to the past. The fourth stage involves letting go and is often a stage of optimism

5 *Testing*: Staff become much more active, trying out new behaviours and ways of coping with the transition and change

6 *Search for meaning*: There is much more understanding of the changes needed within the organization. Once staff have understood how the changes affect their roles within the organization, they are able to move to the final stage

7 *Internalization*: The changes are accepted and become part of daily routine and practice. At this point, staff become more positive, and begin to build on the new strengths they have developed

Developmental, transitional, and transformational change

Barr and Dowding (2012) and Iles and Sutherland (2001) identify three kinds of change:

1 Developmental change
2 Transitional change
3 Transformational change

Developmental change

Developmental change can be seen to improve the effectiveness of current practice within the organization – for example, the focus of change could be the implementation of care bundles (discussed further in Chapter 7) and the skills and processes required to implement care bundles. It can either be planned (deliberate) or emergent (sometimes unfolds in a natural, spontaneous, and unplanned way) (Iles and Sutherland, 2001).

Planned change may occur as a result of external political, economic, social, or technical factors impacting on the organization (Mullins, 2010). These external factors would be clearly demonstrated using a PEST analysis. This change may occur because of an intended change by the change agent, and therefore leaders, as the change agents in healthcare, need to think about and plan the changes carefully. They must ensure that the change occurs at the right time, is relevant, and impacts positively on staff, patients, and service users alike. If leaders communicate and involve staff, patients, and service users in this planned change, there is likely to be less resistance (Iles and Sutherland, 2001; Barr and Dowding, 2012).

Emergent change could be seen as a more bottom-up approach where front-line staff constantly problem-solve together, implementing a range of solutions (Parkin, 2009), and therefore the change takes place automatically.

Transitional change

Transitional change involves the implementation of something different (Figure 4.2). It can be episodic, planned, or a radical organizational change, such as, for example, the move in the UK in April 2013 from Primary Care Trusts to Clinical Commissioning Groups, who are now the commissioners of most National Health Services in England. Management of the interim transition state is needed over a controlled period of time (Iles and Sunderland, 2001; Barr and Dowding, 2012), as staff will be going through the stages of transition as outlined in Figure 4.1.

Transformational change

Transformational change is the emergence of a new state, unknown until it takes shape (Figure 4.3). The time taken for this change is not easily controlled and involves a major change of structures, processes, and the culture within an organization (Iles and Sunderland, 2001; Barr and Dowding, 2012).

For example, the accident and emergency team may identify that having an acute admissions unit would improve patient experience. The introduction

Figure 4.2 Transitional change

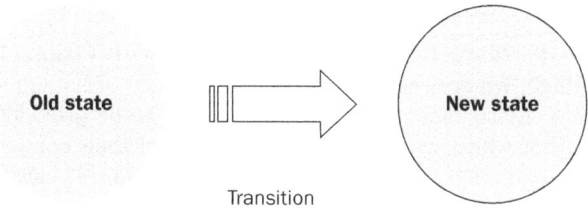

Adapted from: Iles and Sutherland (2001: 16).

Figure 4.3 Transformational change

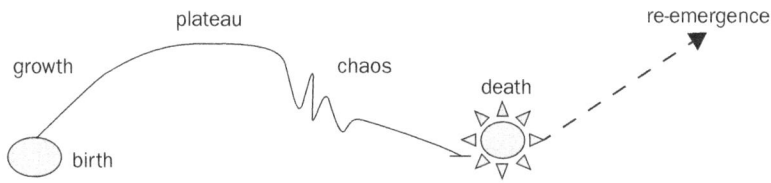

Adapted from: Iles and Sutherland (2001: 16).

of an acute admissions unit linked to the accident and emergency department but functioning as a separate department could help reduce the four-hour waiting time. The new acute admissions unit would act as a gateway between the GP, the emergency department, and the wards of the hospital and therefore improve collaboration. However, for this to happen, consideration would need to be given to the structures, processes, and culture within the organization.

Whatever the nature of the change, Kotter and Schlesinger (2008) suggest there are three key steps to implementing successful change, which any model of change must accommodate:

1 Analysing the situational factors
2 Agreeing the most favourable pace of change
3 Considering how resistance to change will be managed

Key points

- Change may be planned or emergent
- Change may be episodic or radical
- It can take time to adapt to new changes

Leadership and the management of change

If we return to the first definition of clinical governance in Chapter 1 (Department of Health, 1998), we are reminded of the importance of having standards and promoting an environment to enable quality care to be provided. There is an expectation that whilst working within the limits of their competence, health-care professionals such as nurses, midwives, and nursing associates will ensure that their practice is evidence-based and the safety of patients is considered paramount. There is also an expectation that standards of practice will be adhered to (NMC, 2015). Examples of other professional bodies that concur with the Nursing and Midwifery Council (NMC) code are The Chartered Society of Physiotherapists (CSP, 2019), the Royal College of Occupational Therapists (RCOT, 2015), and the Health & Care Professions Council (HCPC, 2014).

We have discussed the fact that management of change can be both invigorating and challenging and yet it is an essential part of healthcare practice. We have discussed that change may be planned or emergent, developmental, transitional, or transformational. However, what is key to health and social care professionals implementing and managing change and adhering to their codes of practice is good leadership. It is important to remember that we can all be good leaders and do not necessarily need to be in a senior position of leadership to be a leader.

Having said that all practitioners can be good leaders, good leadership needs to begin at the senior levels of an organization. Brown (2020) carried out research focusing on the importance of communication and leadership in applying clinical governance strategies to achieving quality healthcare provision. Using a stratified sampling approach, she conducted a comparative case study involving eight Australian public hospitals. Semi-structured interviews and observations were used to collect data from seven CEOs, 15 board members, and 17 senior managers who had responsibility and were accountable for the quality of healthcare provided. A document review was also undertaken: "Questions explored board quality committee processes and characteristics of leadership and communication" (Brown, 2020: 14), resulting in a number of case studies being identified.

Results demonstrated that board members and senior managers could increase staff engagement with the application of clinical governance through key aspects of open communication and leadership. Managers need to be aware that when presenting information around healthcare quality issues, a clear account needs to be given to board members and board members need to challenge managers in a constructive way so that they can gain a broader assessment of the issues. These open discussions enable senior members of an organization time to reflect on the effectiveness of the application of clinical governance, and from this they can identify what learning opportunities and development need to be provided to facilitate successful change. Shared and aligned leadership between CEOs and the board chair was also likely to lead to staff engagement with healthcare governance because they had a shared vision related to the importance of quality healthcare provision.

In the Republic of Ireland, purposeful sampling was used to identify and interview 25 senior managers from five mental health services who had experience of organizational change and who also had been involved in organizational restructuring (Frawley, Meehan, and De Brun, 2018). Senior leaders included the Head of Occupational Therapy, Principal Social Worker, Principal Psychologist, Director of Nursing, Director of Human Resources, and Head of Mental Health. Results demonstrated that leadership and accountability were key to engaging and empowering staff to be involved in changing practice to ensure patient safety. Sharing of information and open communication was also key when implementing change, highlighting similarities with Brown's (2020) research.

If organizational change is going to be successful and levels of patient safety are to be improved, good leadership is required at the very top. As well as communicating with CEOs, senior leaders need to meet with frontline staff to gain an understanding of what is happening and to show that the changes frontline staff are making are important and are leading to greater patient safety. Having a culture of continuous quality improvement (CQI) and management of resistance is key; however, this can be seen to be complex and difficult when organizational change includes merging of teams who may have different cultural norms. If professional teams are going to be merged, further education is required to ensure inter-professional recognition. If change fatigue is to be avoided, clear evidence-based strategies are also essential to manage continuous change and ensure retention of staff within mental health organizations.

Although both of the above studies gathered qualitative data with small sample sizes, what is evident is that good leadership needs to begin at the top of an organization and that future and current leaders throughout the organization need to be supported.

One example of how leaders can be supported is through a leadership academy. As part of NHS England and Improvement, the NHS Leadership Academy provides face-to-face and online courses at local levels to support the development of both new and experienced leaders (NHS Leadership Academy, 2013), so frontline staff who are not in a management position as well as those who are can be helped to develop their leadership skills.

Activity 4.6

Whilst you may not work within the NHS or the UK, the following link will help develop ideas in relation to developing your leadership skills:

https://www.leadershipacademy.nhs.uk/resources/healthcare-leadership-model/ (accessed: 7 March 2021)

The NHS Leadership Academy (2013) has developed a Healthcare Leadership Model to empower and enable healthcare professionals to develop their leadership skills. This model discusses nine dimensions and those leadership behaviours that leaders in healthcare need to demonstrate. Now:

- Go through each dimension and decide which part of the scale relates to you.
- Are you strong in some, exemplary in others, essential or proficient in still others?
- Consider your strengths as well as which areas you could develop.

If you work within primary care and want to read further, you can download the NHS leadership Academy e-book on the following link:

https://www.leadershipacademy.nhs.uk/ (accessed: 7 March 2021)

Activity 4.7

Access the following link:

https://www.england.nhs.uk/wp-content/uploads/2018/03/leadership-development.pdf (accessed: 7 March 2021)

This document facilitates understanding of key aspects related to leadership for Integrated Urgent Care service employers and employees. It also refers to the healthcare leadership model you accessed above (NHS England and Health Education England, 2018), and includes further links of where those working in the UK can access leadership programmes.

There are a number of leadership styles that individuals can choose to adopt but it is not the remit of this book to discuss these in any depth. Lumbers suggests that in particular transformational and democratic leadership styles can lead to successful change management: "These approaches value and empower others' opinions while enabling the team to participate in decision making and providing ownership of the project" (2018: 557).

Key points

- Good leadership is needed for the successful management of change
- Clear, open communication between leaders and frontline staff is essential
- All leaders, regardless of whether they are senior management or frontline staff, need to be supported and encouraged to take part in a leadership development programme

Models of change

There are a number of models that could be used within change management to support leaders and teams applying the principles of clinical governance. Five will be discussed here:

1 Diffusion of Innovation theory
2 RAID
3 Lewin's Force-Field Analysis
4 Kotter's 8-Step Process
5 The Four A's of change

Regardless of the change model chosen, there are three basic aspects that it must consider:

• Recognition of the need to change
• Implementation of an action plan for change (goals and strategies)
• A period of consolidation and evaluation

Diffusion of Innovation model of change

Diffusion is defined as the "process by which an innovation is communicated through certain channels over time among members of a social system. It is a special type of communication, in that the messages are concerned with new ideas" (Rogers, 1983: 5).

At a simplistic level, this is about the ways that are used to communicate new ideas and changes to practice. If the idea is perceived by change agents (policy-makers, leaders, and managers) as being new, it is considered an innovation. When innovative ideas are adopted and diffused, resulting in outcomes, social change has transpired (Rogers, 1983). This model works in two ways in that healthcare teams may adopt the change but then decide to revert to the original practice, or may initially reject the proposed change but then adopt it at a later date. Rogers (1983, cited in Sullivan and Garland, 2013: 195) identifies five steps to this model:

1 *Knowledge*: The proposed change is communicated to staff so that they have an understanding of the change and rationale behind the change
2 *Persuasion*: Staff may be either for or against the proposed change
3 *Decision*: Teams collaborate and discuss the change in order either to adopt or not adopt it
4 *Implementation*: The new change is implemented and the strengths and limitations of the innovation evaluated. Further changes may occur following evaluation
5 *Confirmation*: If the innovation is considered positive and successful following evaluation, change continues, otherwise the innovation is rejected. If unsuccessful, the innovator may decide to review the initiative and implement it at a later date

Table 4.1 Critique of the Diffusion of Innovation model

Strengths	Limitations
• Focuses on new ideas and innovative practice • Allows flexibility in adoption or rejection of proposed innovative change • Allows teams to progress through stages before final adoption of the innovation • Recognizes that equal numbers of individuals are either for or against adopting the change • If change is rejected, the model allows the innovator to make alterations to proposed change and revive the innovation	• Requires commitment and support of policy-makers, leaders, and managers • Getting a new idea adopted is difficult due to uncertainty • Adopting innovations can be a lengthy process • Requires effective and clear two-way communication

Adapted from: Rogers (1983), Sullivan and Garland (2013).

Sullivan and Garland (2013) identify one disadvantage of this model in that it is imperative for the innovators to have the support of policy-makers, leaders, and managers within the organization, because without this the proposed change is unlikely to succeed.

According to Rogers, in the main these five steps must occur in a "… time-ordered sequence of knowledge, persuasion, decision, implementation, and confirmation. The innovation–decision period is the length of time required to pass through the innovation–decision period process" (1983: 21).

Table 4.1 identifies some strengths and limitations of the Diffusion of Innovation model.

We have already discussed how some individuals are enthusiastic and adopt any change quickly and in a positive manner, whereas others are more resistant to change and take longer to adopt new processes, structures, and procedures. Table 4.2 illustrates how Rogers (1983) uses a specific system for classifying adopters, based on the time it takes to adopt new, innovative ideas.

Activity 4.8

Refer back to the first activity in this chapter where you reflected on a change that occurred in your organization. Questions for you to think about include:

• Would you consider this change to be innovative? Reflect on the rationale for your answer.
• In your organization and/or team, who would you consider to be the innovators, early adopters, or early majority?

- Was this change successfully implemented due to the innovators, early adopters, or early majority?
- What did these early adopters do to make the change process smooth and successful?
- In your organization and/or team, who would you consider to be the late majority and laggards?
- Did the late majority and laggards impact on the implementation of the change?
- Why did these late adopters resist the change?

Table 4.2 The five categories of adopters

Innovators	A minority 2–3% of the population who are in the higher socio-economic group, who try out and adopt new ideas quickly. Although they may be regarded as capricious and not be trusted in the decisions by the majority of the community, they may be able to influence the next group
Early adopters	The 10–20% of the population who have a significant role within their community. They are more predisposed to change and have the means, whether personal, social, or financial, to take on board innovation and therefore are more likely to have an influence on the rest of the community
Early majority	They form the 30–35% of the population who are more willing to change and are also won over to the idea of change being the right thing. However, although a larger percentage of the population, they are not in positions than enable them to influence early adopters
Late majority	Also form 30–35% of the population and tend to be sceptics who doubt new ideas until their worth has been clearly demonstrated
Laggards	The 10–20% of the population that tends to be from homogeneous, isolated groups. The most cautious group who are obdurate in accepting change and may not adopt new ideas at all

Adapted from: Rogers (1983).

The RAID model of change

The RAID model (Review, Agreement, Implementation, and Demonstration; Figure 4.4) has been used within UK NHS organizations successfully and was developed by the National Clinical Governance Support Team (Bull and Veall, 2009). According to Rogers, "the experiences of patients and staff have been

Figure 4.4 The RAID model

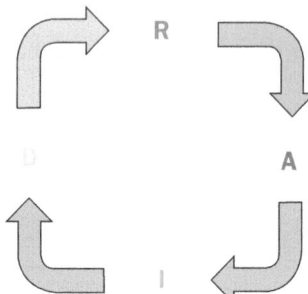

Adapted from: Rogers (2006: 74).

improved by the teams who have used the RAID approach to bring about change" (2006: 79).

According to Rogers (2006) and Bull and Veall (2009), the strengths of this cyclical model are that:

- It allows creativity and innovation and facilitates a bottom-up approach
- It fosters continuous education and training of staff to enable and motivate them to maintain continuous changes to their practice

RAID is based on the acceptance that those who are delivering and managing healthcare services, as well as those receiving healthcare services, are involved in the decision-making. This therefore differs from a top-down hierarchical approach. This does not mean that managers should not be included – indeed their support is vital. A change initiative such as the implementation of clinical governance strategies is more likely to be effective if managers, ward managers, frontline staff, patients, and service users communicate and collaborate. However, involvement in decision-making is not sufficient and Bull and Veall (2009) emphasize that another advantage of this model is that it fosters ongoing education and training of staff to enable and motivate them to maintain continuous changes to their practice. Figure 1.4 (page 17) illustrates how education and training are a key clinical governance strategy.

In order to review the challenges and achievements and implement any change process, good communication skills and listening skills are vital (Bishop, 2010) during all stages of this model.

Stage 1: Review

The first stage of the model involves a working group to review the current service both at a local and national level. This review involves the gathering of information from those in management positions, clinical and non-clinical staff, service users, carers, and families (Rogers, 2006), and therefore supports the definition of service user involvement (Seden *et al.*, 2010) that we discussed in Chapter 1. One of the advantages of having such a varied group is that those who are directly affected by the change can be involved from the beginning. They can share their experiences of the current service provision and can also have a say in any planned changes, thus having a "sense of ownership" (Rogers, 2006: 5). This supports the notion that RAID is a bottom-up model of change. The final part of this stage is for the team to suggest potential recommendations demonstrating how changes and improvements to the quality of service provision will be achieved.

Stage 2: Agree

During this stage of this model, the review panel agrees on specific actions and changes. Those at the top of the organization and those involved in the review need to be confident that the proposed changes support the organization's strategic direction. Managers have to ensure that any changes to the service do not negatively impact on other services. At a more local level, teams will have to ensure that changes are prioritized and operationalized. It is not always possible to implement all recommendations at the same time, and therefore teams will have to prioritize and perhaps select changes that are easy to implement successfully without too many resources (Rogers, 2006).

Stage 3: Implement

This stage involves recommendations being actioned and requires strong leadership. Leaders need to identify the agenda, timetable, and actions required in order to implement the recommendations (Rogers, 2006). Barr and Dowding (2012) suggest that a Gannt chart (developed by Gannt in the early twentieth century), commonly used within healthcare practice and easily downloaded from the internet, be used to draw up this timetable.

Stage 4: Demonstrate

As with all models of change, this stage involves evaluation. If some aspects of the change process are deemed to have been unsuccessful, teams can discuss lessons learned and reflect on actions to be taken to develop current strategies. It is essential that the results of the evaluation are disseminated to the members of the original review group as well as the employees of the organization. Patients and service users may wish to communicate successful changes using the Patient Voices Programme mentioned in Chapter 1.

Worked example from practice: diabetes care

Figure 4.5 illustrates how the RAID model was used in practice to increase the number of link-nurses working with individuals with diabetes as well as working with secondary care nurses, their families and carers. We can see that the key clinical governance strategy implemented in this worked example is education and training and this strategy will be discussed in more depth in the next chapter.

Aims of project

- To increase the number and motivation of secondary care link-nurses within the district general hospital site
- To enhance their knowledge and bridge the theory–practice gap in dissemination of that knowledge (Bull and Veall, 2009)

In this worked example, the application of the RAID model was successful because:

- A bottom-up approach was used
- Support for link-nurses was provided through education and training

Figure 4.5 RAID, worked example from practice: diabetes care

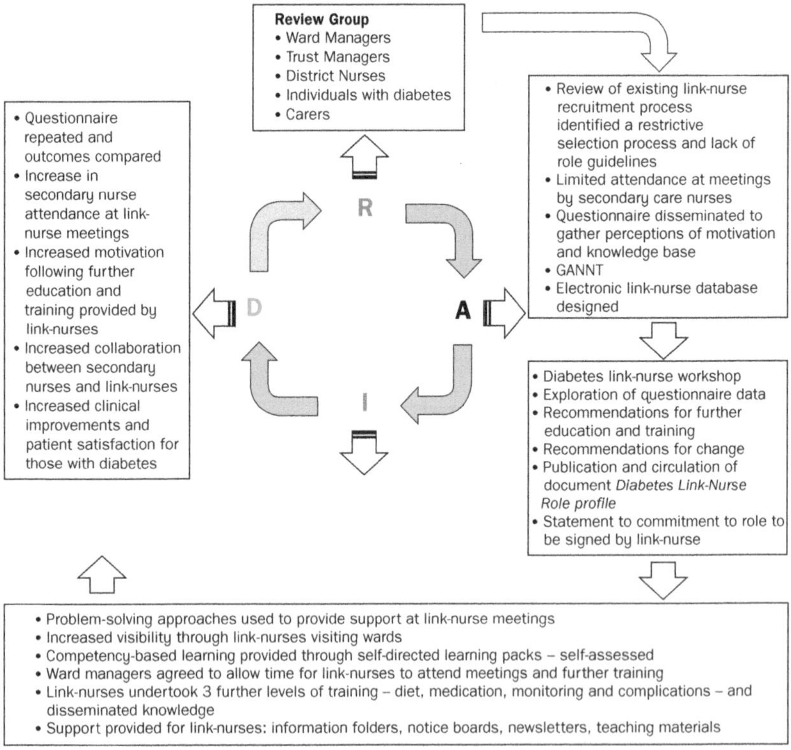

Review Group
- Ward Managers
- Trust Managers
- District Nurses
- Individuals with diabetes
- Carers

- Questionnaire repeated and outcomes compared
- Increase in secondary nurse attendance at link-nurse meetings
- Increased motivation following further education and training provided by link-nurses
- Increased collaboration between secondary nurses and link-nurses
- Increased clinical improvements and patient satisfaction for those with diabetes

R

D

A

I

- Review of existing link-nurse recruitment process identified a restrictive selection process and lack of role guidelines
- Limited attendance at meetings by secondary care nurses
- Questionnaire disseminated to gather perceptions of motivation and knowledge base
- GANNT
- Electronic link-nurse database designed

- Diabetes link-nurse workshop
- Exploration of questionnaire data
- Recommendations for further education and training
- Recommendations for change
- Publication and circulation of document *Diabetes Link-Nurse Role profile*
- Statement to commitment to role to be signed by link-nurse

- Problem-solving approaches used to provide support at link-nurse meetings
- Increased visibility through link-nurses visiting wards
- Competency-based learning provided through self-directed learning packs – self-assessed
- Ward managers agreed to allow time for link-nurses to attend meetings and further training
- Link-nurses undertook 3 further levels of training – diet, medication, monitoring and complications – and disseminated knowledge
- Support provided for link-nurses: information folders, notice boards, newsletters, teaching materials

Adapted from: Bull and Veall (2009).

- This increased their knowledge in relation to diabetes care
- The impact of this was that these link-nurses were able to disseminate their knowledge to nurses involved in the care of those with diabetes
- This in turn led to improved care and service user/patient satisfaction

---

Key points

- RAID involves managers, frontline staff, patients, and carers
- RAID is a bottom-up approach
- RAID facilitates change and improves service delivery and quality care

---

Activity 4.9

Consider your own area of practice.

- Reflect on your target population and choose one group, for example stroke, substance misuse.
- Consider an issue where the quality of care could be improved for this group.
- Refer back to Figure 4.4 and, taking each stage in turn (review, agreement, implementation, and demonstration), consider how this model could be used to manage the change process and resolve your quality issue.
- Who would you involve in the review group?
- How could you go about applying this model to practice?

Table 4.3 identifies some strengths and limitations of the RAID model.

Table 4.3   Critique of the RAID model

Strengths	Limitations
• A bottom-up model • Engages service users and staff in quality improvement programmes • Identifies key projects for teams to engage with • Allows creativity and innovation (Rogers, 2006) • Encourages problem-solving • Motivates staff to continually develop the quality of healthcare provision • Fosters continuous professional development through education and training	• Too many recommendations made by the review panel may be unachievable • Requires resources to provide education and training to staff in order for changes to be implemented

Lewin's Force-Field Analysis model of change

Lewin (1951, cited in Sale, 2005) discusses using a Force-Field Analysis (Figure 4.6) and describes the notion of examining the forces at work and manipulating any or all of these forces to achieve change. In order for this analysis to work, there needs to be a movement in thinking. Lewin describes this as taking place over three stages:

1 Unfreezing
2 Change
3 Refreezing

Unfreezing

During the unfreezing stage, participants in the process will acknowledge that change is necessary and that current systems/processes require changing. The proposed changes may include an assessment of the current situation, for example a change in:

* The organization
* Management
* Practice

Once assessment has taken place, an action plan will be instigated.

Change

An acknowledgement that change is required will enable the use of a Force-Field Analysis during the change stage of Lewin's model. This analysis can take place only if unfreezing occurs. The Force-Field Analysis shows how change can be aided by reducing resistive forces effectively while progressively

Figure 4.6 Lewin's Force-Field Analysis model

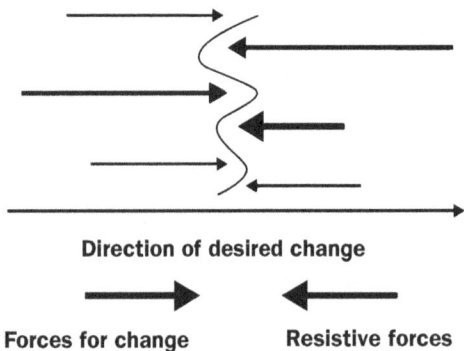

Direction of desired change

Forces for change   **Resistive forces**

Adapted from: Lewin (1953), cited in Sale (2005).

increasing the driving forces (Swage, 2004). The resisting and driving forces are identified by the respective arrows in Figure 4.6. The thickness of the arrows highlights the strength of the resistor or driver; the thicker the arrow, the stronger the force.

Refreezing

Refreezing occurs when the action plan has been implemented, the changes in practice become the norm, and the quality of care improved because the drivers have been strengthened and the resistors weakened.

Worked example from practice: medication errors

If we return to the worked example using Ishikawa's fishbone analysis of medication errors discussed in Chapter 3 (Figure 3.4; page 56), we can see a number of causes identified by the team that could be used to explain the reasons leading to medication errors.

In order to facilitate any change and improvement in quality care, the next stage for the team could be to use their initial analysis and identify the key drivers and resistors linked to medication errors; the beginning of this analysis is shown in Figure 4.7.

Having added the thick and thin arrows (drivers and resistors), the next stage for the team will be to consider which clinical governance strategies could be used to reduce the resistors and strengthen the drivers.

Figure 4.7 Force-Field Analysis for medication errors

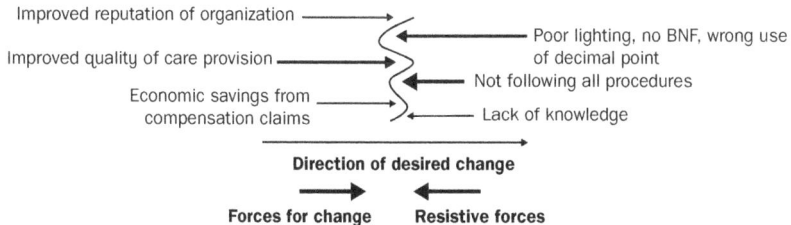

Activity 4.10

Refer back to Figure 1.4 (page 17), the framework of clinical governance. Which clinical governance strategies (EBP, research and development, education and training, risk management, complaints management or audit) could be considered in order that the resistors could be reduced and drivers strengthened?

You may have considered risk management because of the poor lighting, no BNF, and wrong use of decimal point. You may also have considered education and training due to the lack of knowledge, as well as audit to measure the change in practice and reduction of medication errors and financial

Table 4.4 Critique of Lewin's Force-Field analysis model

Strengths	Limitations
• It is a simple tool • It is easy to understand and use • Helps teams identify the strengths of resistors to and drivers of change • Helps teams to prioritize resistors and drivers through the thickness of arrows • Only has a few steps for teams to follow	• It is only part of Lewin's wider Planned Approach to Change, and is therefore somewhat simplistic, as discussed in further detail below

compensation costs. These clinical governance strategies will be discussed in Chapters 5 and 6.

Table 4.4 identifies some strengths and limitations of Lewin's Force-Field analysis model.

Kotter's 8-Step Process model of change

According to Kotter (2012), organizations need competent managers but also leaders of change: 70–90% of change occurs because of good leadership, whereas 10–30% of change occurs due to good management. Kotter (2012) discusses how leaders need to define what the future will look like. They need to support people to enable them to understand the vision for the future, thus motivating and enthusing them to make the changes regardless of barriers and obstacles with which they might be faced.

Steps 1–4 below show how leaders can support staff and reduce the status quo within the organization. Steps 5–7 are taken to introduce new practices and the final Step 8 occurs when the changes to practice are consolidated and become part of the organizational culture. It is essential that all eight steps are followed because, if not, it is less likely that the changes in practice will be long-lasting or successful. It is also essential that staff are not made to feel pressurized into moving onto the next step too soon. Much of the onus is on good leaders, however, they also need to be supported so they can engage in lifelong learning. Lifelong learning will be discussed in more depth in the following chapter.

Over the years, many countries have moved from paper-based patient records to electronic medical records, including the UK (Electronic Health Record: EHR), Canada (Electronic Medical Records: EMR), Hong Kong (Inpatient Medication Entry Order System: IPMOE), Europe (Electronic Health Records: EMR), China (Electronic Medical Records: EMR), USA (Electronic Health Records: EHR), Africa (Electronic Health Records: EHR), and Australia (Personally Controlled Electronic Health Record: PCEHR). However, there is some evidence that this change has been met with resistance, an example of which is provided below.

Table 4.5 Kotter's 8-Step Process model of change

Establish a sense of urgency	Healthcare professionals must not become complacent; those with power and credibility (i.e. leaders) need to ensure that all staff are supported in order to implement changes within practice. Investigations and reports following incidences identified in Chapter 1, such as Winterbourne View and poor quality care within mental health services, made clear recommendations for change. Leaders need to identify future possible crises and major opportunities such as those faced by staff during the 2020–2021 world pandemic
Create the guiding coalition	Leaders with sufficient power need to be able to bring teams together. For this to happen, all staff need to have trust in their leaders and be supported to keep pace with change. Again, this can be linked to the COVID-19 pandemic where staff in intensive care units had to rapidly adjust to changes in practice
Develop a vision and strategy	Leaders need to ensure staff understand the vision and clarify any misconceptions about the future. Additionally, they need to motivate staff and coordinate actions needed to implement successful change
Communicate the change vision	Leaders need to ensure that messages given are consistent and more importantly make sure that all messages are communicated clearly and succinctly. This is not an easy undertaking
Empower broad-based action	Staff at all levels need to feel empowered to undertake the required changes. Management must employ the right staff – this was one of the failings identified at Winterbourne View (discussed in Chapter 1)
Generate short-term wins	The successful beginnings of change (short-term wins) and successful results are the motivating factor to continue for the long term
Consolidate gains and produce more change	Staff cannot become complacent once short-term wins are identified. Leaders need to continue to keep rewards and the transformation of change going. They need to continue to reduce the resistors and maintain a sense of urgency such as seen in worldwide ICUs during the 2020 pandemic
Anchor new approaches in the culture	Lastly, leaders need to continue to motivate all staff so that a change in the culture of the organization is maintained with shared values and norms

Auguste (2013) conducted some research because the implementation of electronic medical records (EMR) and conversion to a fully digital clinic was not supported by a group of orthopaedic surgeons and their staff in a practice group in Toronto despite the Ontario Medical Association's requirement and funding to do so. Kotter's 8-Step Process for Leading Change was used to support the transformation.

- The paper-based tasks used by the surgeons and staff were identified
- The digital alternatives using an EMR were implemented
- Kotter's 8-Step Process for Leading Change was administered, leading to a 95%+ adoption of an EMR

Eight of the 10 staff (three surgeons and five administrators) took part in pre-adoption interviews to investigate attitudes to change, and qualitative open coding was used to analyse the data. At the start of each interview, the researcher outlined the need for change and how Kotter's model would be employed. The researcher asked two questions:

1 Why do you continue to use paper-based processes when digital alternatives are available?
2 What are the residual paper-based processes that you currently use?

The following staff member perceived barriers were identified using a narrative analysis of the interview data:

Expressed barrier	Frequency of mention
Lack of knowledge of digital alternatives	100% (8/8)
Habit	75% (6/8)
Lack of motivation to change	50% (4/8)
Lack of knowledge of consequences	50% (4/8)

Each step in Kotter's model was discussed with each participant (see Table 4.6).

Table 4.7 identifies some strengths and limitations of Kotter's 8-Step Process model of change.

Before discussing the next model, it is useful to compare Lewin's Force-Field Analysis and Kotter's 8-Step Process:

- Lewin's theory is based on a simple roadmap: Unfreeze, Change, Refreeze. Kotter's eight steps are not so simple
- Lewin's theory appears more logical (think about the placement of Step 3 in Kotter's theory) and therefore might be easier for those new to the management of change to understand and utilize
- Lewin's model is based on human psychology (Lewin was a psychologist), focusing on behaviours that block and drive change. Kotter's model is less concerned with behaviours, apart from being motivated and the urgency for change

Table 4.6 Worked example: electronic medical records

Kotter's 8-Step Process for leading change	
Step 1: *Communicate urgency*	The Ontario Medical Association's deadline for support and funding were emphasized
Step 2: *Build a guiding team*	A physician champion and an administrative champion were elected to communicate the vision and act as role models
Step 3: *Create a vision*	Face-to-face meetings, email reminders, electronic feedback from the EMR programme to demonstrate functionality, familiarity, and ease of use
Step 4: *Communicate for buy-in*	Face-to-face meetings, email reminders, electronic feedback from the EMR programme to demonstrate functionality, familiarity, and ease of use
Step 5: *Remove obstacles*	One-to-one in-house training on the EMR programme; one-to-one support from the researcher
Step 6: *Create short-term wins to provide momentum*	Meeting between the physician champion and OntarioMD (the company supporting physician practices in the selection, implementation, and adoption of EMRs) and final approval of grant funding for the adoption of EMR use
Step 7: *Maintain momentum*	Confirmation of adoption from OntarioMD and confirmation of digital integration between the practice and the hospital
Step 8: *Incorporate change into organizational culture*	Adoption of digital process will be supported by email and monthly staff meetings. The ceremonial shredding of paper forms was celebrated at a major clinic social event

Adapted from: Auguste (2013).

- Despite the lack of *how* the steps might be accomplished, Kotter's model does give more detail than Lewin's. And whilst Lewin's model is simple, it might be considered too simple. Perhaps there is a case for combining the two models

Bird (2020) supports the case for adopting both of the above models when using change management to increase adherence to the use of barcode medicines administration technology. Despite the use of barcode administration, patient misidentification leading to medication errors continues to occur and can result in serious harm to patients (Hospital Authority Hong Kong, 2021; CQC, 2018; Song, Park, and Oh, 2015).

"The Global Digital Exemplar (GDE) programme is a knowledge-sharing platform developed by NHS England that aims to deliver quality of care through digital technologies and information" (Bird, 2020). These exemplars are internationally recognized. However, in England, in order to be given funding from this GDE programme, hospitals must use barcode medicine administration technology. The *Five Year Forward View* (NHS, 2014) and *The NHS Long Term Plan* (NHS, 2019) (see Chapter 1) both state that if hospitals continue to be paper-based, they are less likely to embrace new technologies such as barcode medicine administration.

Bird (2020) discusses how Kotter's 8-Step Process model was used to guide the pilot stage of a programme of change implemented with the aim of increasing compliance with the use of barcode administration technology (sense of urgency). Three wards took part in this pilot project. Staff in two of the wards checked patients' identification by their beds and the medication was kept in a separate room. The team in the third ward decided to change their trolleys to ones that were large enough to include a computer. This resulted in greater staff compliance and was considered one of Kotter's small wins. Following this pilot phase, Lewin's 1951 model was used to manage a wider application and use of barcode technology across all wards. It can be seen that the status quo of the Trust was the low compliance with use of the barcode technology. With a view to changing practice and increasing staff compliance, the unfreezing stage was officially launched by instigating the compulsory use of larger medicine trolleys incorporating computers throughout the Trust. The refreezing stage and standardization of practice became the norm.

Although compliance did improve, there were differing results across the wards, which Bird (2020) puts this down to the impact that leaders can also have on the adoption process.

Table 4.7 Critique of Kotter's 8-Step Process for change model

Strengths	Limitations
• Identifies a step-by-step process for leaders and teams to follow • Steps are logical, clear, and easy to follow • The importance of getting help is emphasized • The importance of motivating staff is also emphasized • The model is instinctive • Supports transformational change • Promotes team engagement • Short-term wins can be motivating • Supports the culture of the organization to become one that shares values and norms	• Could be seen to lack flexibility • Steps must be followed in order • Eight steps might be seen by some as too many • Prescriptive • Not a suitable model to apply to all situations, for example, COVID-19 when the response to patient care was urgent • Lacks detail on how steps might be accomplished, for example by using a change impact assessment • Steps might appear to be out of order; for example, does it not make more sense for Step 3 to become Step 1? • It could be seen as a top-down approach focusing on urgency and removing barriers to motivation rather than focusing on employees

The Four A's model of change

Focusing on change in a healthcare setting, Barrett (2003) discussed a four-stage process of change, whether macro or micro, which he identified as the Four A's of change:

1 Antecedence
2 Analysis of options
3 Action on change
4 Aftermath of change

Stage 1: Antecedence

This part of the process involves identifying the need for change, and Barrett (2003) suggests the following seven prompts:

1 *Awakening*: realizing that there are challenges to the status quo
2 *Reactionary*: includes an increase in patient/user complaints
3 *Imposition hierarchy*: top-down imposed change
4 *Inverted hierarchy*: bottom-up request for change
5 *Maturation*: evolution of the individual or organization
6 *Adaptation*: changes to procedures or processes
7 *Invention*: keeping abreast of changes in technology, drugs, surgical techniques, and so on

Antecedence is key to the process of change, as opposition to change will be reduced if there is an understanding of why change is required. Barrett (2003) suggests that situational analysis is an important part of antecedence, as it looks at the current situation. He suggests the use of two simple tools, SWOT and PESTLE (Mullins, 2010), which are discussed in greater detail in Chapter 3.

Stage 2: Analysis of options

The next stage in the process is a considered analysis of options and the communication of these to the decision-makers involved in the change process. For this to take place effectively, there needs to be an "intention to act" (Barrett, 2003: 154). Having choice – that is, a number of options – can result in uncertainty and decision-makers need to be aware of this and be able to cope with possible dilemmas in order to achieve the desired change. There is an extensive literature concerning decision-making, but this will not be discussed here.

Stage 3: Action on change

Identifying problem areas and opportunities for change is often the remit of one or more individuals who Barrett (2003) refers to as change agents. That is, someone "who identifies major problem areas, identifies the opportunities for change, builds readiness and commitment, builds a renewing system through creating a climate for change and establishes internal capacity to sustain the change effort, evaluate it and review it" (Broome, 1998: 87).

A change agent may be internal or external to an organization, depending on the required change, and must motivate and deal with conflict as the proposed change is being discharged. Cahill (1995) describes three types of change agent:

1 *Adopters* hear about successful change and incorporate it into their practice (note the synergy with Roger's (1983) term in his Classification of Adopters, discussed earlier)
2 *Generators* motivate and change attitudes
3 *Implementers* initiate change once a decision to change has been recognized by generators

It is widely agreed that, in order to implement change, a theoretical approach needs to be taken and many would use Lewin's three-step change at this stage of the process. This is the case with Barrett (2003), who uses the three-step model both simplistically and in isolation.

It is widely believed that Lewin's three-step model is his key contribution to organizational change, but Burnes (2004) argues that Lewin did not intend his model to be used in isolation. What often seems to be forgotten is that Lewin was a humanitarian and his work stemmed from a passion to resolve social conflict, particularly the problems associated with minority or disadvantaged groups. He believed that using a Planned Approach to Change, which includes Field Theory, Group Dynamics, and Action Research, together with the three-step model could bring about change at an individual, group, organzational, and societal level (Burnes, 2004). What seems to have happened is that theorists have unpicked Lewin's Planned Approach to Change, merely focusing on the three-step model. This is highlighted by Hendry, who states, "Scratch any account of creating and managing a change and the idea that change is a three-stage process which necessarily begins with a process of unfreezing will not be far below the surface" (1996: 624). This said, Barrett (2003) does recommend using Lewin's three-step theory as a theoretical approach to change but also calls for the identification of change strategies, focusing on three general strategies:

1 *Rational-empirical strategy*: This is based on the premise that many are guided by self-interest and reason and if they see the proposed change as benefitting them, they will support it. This is normally a top-down approach

2 *Power-coercive strategy*: Also a top-down approach where those in authority instruct others to change

3 *Normative-reductive strategy*: This is a bottom-up approach to change and is values-led. Values and perceptions are altered and new norms are formed

Strategies 1 and 2 may be used where compliance with legal directives is required, for example health and safety legislation, whereas strategy 3 is more appropriate for bringing about social change that benefits all stakeholders, for example patients, carers, and staff.

Whichever of the above strategies is used, the change agent needs to demonstrate good leadership skills. Leaders may be either emergent (the leader is either informally chosen or formally elected by members of the group) or imposed (the leader is appointed or elected by a person or group external to the team to be led) (Sanchez-Cortes *et al.*, 2012) and may adopt one of three leadership styles (Mullins, 2010):

1 Autocratic
2 Democratic
3 Laissez-faire

Tannenbaum and Schmidt (1973, cited in Mullins, 2010) presented a leadership continuum in which leaders may change their style to suit the situation. The categories of leadership in this continuum go from dictatorial to autocratic to democratic to laissez-faire (Figure 4.8). Dictatorial and laissez-faire are extremes in style, with a dictatorial leader making decisions without consultation and the latter unable to make quick and significant decisions.

Democratic leadership (Mullins, 2010) is participative and promotes motivation, productivity, and cohesiveness, and in most change situations would be the leadership style of choice. However, it must be recognized that a democratic form of leadership would not be appropriate in an emergency situation, for example the leadership style required by a nurse coordinating the resuscitation of a patient. Here a dictatorial style would be required.

An integral part of good leadership is the ability to motivate, and there is a plethora of literature on motivation, with early work being undertaken by Maslow (1954), McClelland (1961), and Vroom (1964). All agree that communication is key to motivation, and this is endorsed by Marquis and Huston (1998), who show how leaders use communication to motivate staff to embrace change.

Figure 4.8 A leadership continuum

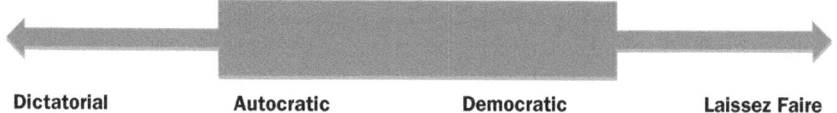

| Dictatorial | Autocratic | Democratic | Laissez Faire |

Implementing change is essential to Barrett's process, and preparation and planning play key roles at this stage. Resistance to change is also natural, but, if managed well, can lead to group cohesion and good group decisions. Gillies (1994) suggests five means of resolving conflict:

1 Competition and power
2 Smoothing
3 Avoidance
4 Compromise
5 Collaboration

Of these, the fifth option is the most suitable in managing change. A collaborative approach to decision-making would involve a recognition that conflict exists, confronting the issues, and collaboratively trying to resolve the issues whilst including all stakeholders in the process.

Stage 4: Aftermath of change

Whatever the change, Barrett (2003) suggests that a contingency plan needs to be in place, which allows a return to the pre-change position if, for whatever reason, the proposed change is unsuccessful. This supports the notion of a trial period of change with the ability to return to the pre-change position if necessary, thus reducing the possibility of fear of failure and risk. And, finally, the process must be evaluated.

To conclude, Barrett (2003) posits that a structured process needs to be in place in order to implement a successful change and that his Four A's provides such. However, there are still some strengths and limitations to this model (Table 4.4).

We have considered above four models that teams could use to facilitate the management of change and each of these models has its strengths and limitations.

Activity 4.11

Reflect on your own practice. Take each model in turn and decide whether you like or dislike the models (Diffusion of Innovation, RAID, Lewin's Force-Field Analysis, Kotter's 8-Step Process, the Four A's).

- What is your rationale for these decisions?
- Can you identify any other strengths and limitations?
- Choose your preferred model.
- Consider an area of practice where the quality of care could be improved.
- Consider how you could apply your preferred model to your practice.

Table 4.8 Critique of Barrett's Four A's model of change

Strengths	Limitations
• Sets out a process for change management, offering four clear steps • Another "bottom-up" model • Engages service users and staff in quality improvement programmes • Motivates staff to continuously develop the quality of healthcare provision by offering a fallback position (contingency plan)	• It uses Lewin's three-step change theory and therefore is somewhat simplistic (as discussed above)

Quality improvement programmes

We have discussed the need for ongoing improvement in the quality of care provided by healthcare staff, and presented five models that teams might find helpful in managing and implementing changes in practice. By embracing management of change, a quality improvement programme can be established.

Jones, Vaux, and Olsson-Brown (2019) discuss some key points to enable healthcare practitioners to engage in a quality improvement programme and therefore clinical governance. First of all, they define quality improvement as follows:

* Quality improvement aims to make a difference to patients by improving safety, effectiveness and experience of care by:
  o Using understanding of our complex healthcare system
  o Applying a systematic approach
  o Designing, testing and implementing changes using real time measurement of improvement. (Jones *et al.*, 2019)

The benefits from these programmes are threefold. First, they aim to improve the quality of patient care but also benefit practitioners and the providers of healthcare. Secondly, planning and developing quality improvement programmes can facilitate healthcare practitioners' skills. For example, by being involved with a quality improvement initiative, their leadership, communication, project management, team working, presentation, and time management skills can be enhanced. And thirdly, these programmes are seen to be empowering and gratifying as well as also facilitating cooperation and collaboration within and across organizations. However, as well as these positive aspects there are also likely to be challenges for those wanting to develop specific practice initiatives, for example staff need to be convinced that there is a specific quality issue, and therefore a need for change, and to feel that they can sustain this change alongside other workplace pressures. Unsupportive management will also impact on the success of any quality improvement programme (Jones *et al.*, 2019).

Jones *et al.* (2019) go on to discuss a number of skills that these leaders of change require, such as "enthusiasm, optimism, curiosity and perseverance". It is also essential that they are able to collaborate with multi- and interdisciplinary teams as well as patients, and they need to have an understanding of the organization's processes and procedures and be able to transform quality improvement methods into practice. The models discussed above might help these leaders.

A quality improvement team needs to be organized and it is important to include both clinical staff and non-clinical staff with a mix of skills. It is beneficial if the leader of this initiative is supported by a colleague with experience of these initiatives (Jones *et al.*, 2019). Once the group is formed, they could form a quality circle (Chapter 3) to brainstorm and identify a specific initiative for change. Data from audits would be useful, as it provides evidence on the need for change (Chapters 3 and 8) and the audit cycle might also be useful to guide the team – that is, identify a problem, gather evidence that there is a problem, agree changes, implement those changes, and finally evaluate the changes. Jones *et al.* (2019) suggest that using a SMART framework (**S**pecific, **M**easurable, **A**chievable, **R**ealistic, and with a **T**imeframe) would guide and focus the agreed quality improvement programme. Alongside this, the team might also include SMART aims and objectives for the programme.

The following discussion will address three specific quality improvement programmes, the first two from the USA and the third from the UK.

Wu *et al.* (2016) explored how an intervention bundle for the discharge process across 11 freestanding tertiary-care children's hospitals could improve the discharge process. It must be noted that community hospitals and general hospitals were not included, and so results cannot be generalized. A SMART aim was agreed, that is: "To reduce discharge-related care failures by 50% in 12 months".

A change package was agreed across these 11 hospitals that included the following:

- Proactive discharge planning throughout the hospitalization
- Improve throughput
- Arrange postdischarge treatment
- Communicate postdischarge plan to providers
- Communicate postdischarge plan to patients and families
- Postdischarge support. (Wu *et al.*, 2016)

The teams were supported by virtual learning sessions and web conferences and in between these sessions the teams implemented small changes. Successes were shared in between these learning sessions and can be likened to Kotter's small wins. Participating units focused on educating families on their child's diagnosis and plans for discharge, written discharge instructions were developed, and in some cases discharge checklists were used. Instructions were made more user-friendly and forms included in electronic medical records. Phone calls using a standardized script were employed as a means to reinforce discharge directives as well as measure any discharge failures. Following the implementation of the discharge plans, a decrease in discharge failures was evident, as was improved communication with families via the post-discharge follow-up calls. However, despite good progress, the 50% SMART aim given above was not achieved (Wu *et al.*, 2016). This highlights the importance when deciding on the percentage for a SMART goal because if it is too high, the goal might not be achieved, and this could make staff feel despondent.

The next example is of a quality improvement programme from Boston, Massachusetts. The case study was published by The Health Foundation (2010), a UK-based organization. Following the merger of two hospitals in Boston, a new CEO was appointed. It became evident that the two hospitals had differing cultures. The merged hospitals were in a financial crisis, the quality and safety of patient care was poor, as was staff morale. Some staff felt disempowered and some chose to leave the organization. The CEO took a strategic approach and implemented a culture of openness and accountability, as he wanted to empower and motivate all clinical and non-clinical staff to engage with improving the quality of care within the organization. This required sound leadership and clinical leaders were appointed as change agents. The CEO was open and honest and made them aware of the financial constraints and problems within the hospital, thus creating a sense of urgency (Step 1 of Kotter's 8-Step Process). These leaders were able to contribute to the operational management of the organization – that is, contribute to how the hospital was run. The CEO listened to staff to gain an understanding of their concerns but also shared his financial concerns with them. The aim was to involve the healthcare professionals to engage with the new hospital's non-clinical objectives and therefore have a better understanding, for example, of the dire financial situation the hospital was in.

To begin with, the focus was on changes within orthopaedic and pancreatic surgery and staff were involved in the operational management of these departments. Staff engaged in the change process and the CEO ensured that he shared the improved patient outcomes, making staff feel proud and giving them a sense that they had accomplished something, leading to increased motivation. This led to further better quality patient outcomes. "Other clinical departments bought into the approach and clinicians started to engage in the design, production and analysis of data" (The Health Foundation, 2010: 11).

There was also a view in the organization that mistakes were just a part of practice. Leaders acknowledged that errors happen and then worked with staff in one particular area to develop their knowledge with regards to the fact that some central line infections were preventable. Once a reduction in infections was achieved, the CEO made this data available to the public via his blog, stating that he was proud of staff who had responded so well. As with the example above, this gave staff a sense of ownership, which led them to become more motivated. Engaging staff in the operational management of the organization led to improved staff morale and better patient outcomes.

The final example comes from the UK. In their paper, Davies, James, and Griffiths (2020) discuss a quality improvement programme established in a

Figure 4.9 Locality driver diagram for the quality improvement programme

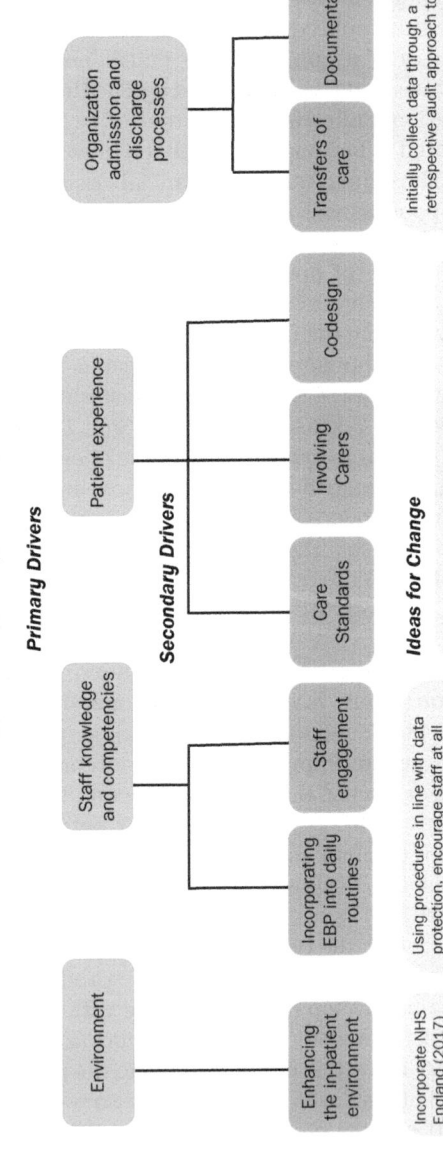

Adapted from: Davies, James and Griffiths (2020).

mental health service in Wales. One idea behind this was that learning from this process could be applied to other Welsh mental health services. Initially, 12 quality improvement multidisciplinary champions were appointed and during 2018 engaged in a number of workshop sessions in order to facilitate their own learning in quality improvement methodology. This group identified drivers for change (as suggested by Lewin, 1951) and also identified areas of practice that needed to be improved and changed, in particular changes that would gain "short-term wins" (Kotter, 2012). These short-term wins helped staff to maintain motivation during times of change. Figure 4.9 above illustrates a number of drivers for change in order for a successful quality improvement programme to be implemented.

***

Activity 4.12

Consider the drivers identified in Figure 4.9.

Using Lewin's Force-Field Analysis, draw a figure showing the drivers from Figure 4.9 and include some resistors for implementing the last quality improvement programme outlined above.

Remember that the arrows used for the drivers and resistors need to vary in thickness because this shows the strength of the driver and resistor.

***

Activity 4.13

In order to develop your learning with regards to *The Fifteen Steps Challenge* (NHS England 2017) identified in Figure 4.9, access the following link.

https://www.england.nhs.uk/wp-content/uploads/2017/11/15-steps-inpatient.pdf (accessed: 7 March 2021)

***

Service user engagement was discussed in Chapter 1. In Davies and colleagues' research (2020), service users and carers were also involved in the quality improvement programme and were given the remit of ensuring that service users, their families and carers were given opportunities to discuss their experience of the mental health service provision. One of the outcomes from this was that it led to an improvement in relationships with healthcare professionals.

Recommendations were made to ensure continued development, one of which was the need to involve a wider group of stakeholders, for example social services. Another key recommendation was to ensure that those leading the change, that is the champions, are continually facilitated to develop and apply their knowledge of quality improvement methodologies.

Quality improvement programmes help to achieve total quality management and therefore must include all grades of staff. When Davies *et al.* (2020) introduced the quality improvement programmes, they did this at ward handovers and staff were given the opportunity to share their experiences. Whilst their article discusses the impact on staff of patient suicide, a further example might include the impact on staff following an outburst of verbal abuse or physical abuse or other such challenging behaviours. These stories were shared digitally, enabling managers to highlight the impact these behaviours might have on staff. It became evident that improving the wellbeing of staff led to an improvement in the quality of care provided. Other areas that improved linked to more accurate electronic transfers of care and fewer readmissions.

This chapter has identified some of the barriers to change and stipulated that change takes time. In their paper, Davies *et al.* (2020) conclude with a recommendation on the importance of celebrating successful changes and using presentations, verbal as well as poster presentations, to illustrate changes within the organization.

Key points summary

In order to improve the quality of care provided within healthcare, managing change and innovation needs to be a constant process. Resistance and uncertainty linked to change and innovation can be expected and therefore a transition phase is important. It is not possible to change everything at one time and if the drivers and resistors are identified, healthcare professionals will be able to prioritize the changes and these can be addressed incrementally.

- It is the healthcare professional's responsibility to raise concerns about quality of care, although this may have repercussions
- Change needs to be collaborative – that is, patients, carers, and staff should be involved in any decision to change and in the change management process
- Change needs to follow a process
- A number of change management models can be utilized to drive the change initiative
- A mix of change management models can be helpful
- Quality improvement programmes facilitate the provision of quality patient care and safety as well as developing skills amongst leaders and teams
- Quality improvement programmes can give staff a sense of ownership, making them feel more empowered, motivated, and committed

Implications for practice

- Any one of the five models for change may be used to facilitate change in a healthcare setting. All have their strengths and limitations and these need to be taken into consideration when adopting a model

- With an understanding of the Diffusion of Innovations model, if you are an early adopter remember to support team members who are either late adopters or laggards
- Change takes time and therefore needs to be supported by management adopting appropriate leadership styles
- Quality improvement initiatives facilitate teams working together to improve quality healthcare provision

End-of-chapter questions

1 What are the main barriers to change?
2 Why does change need to be collaborative?
3 How do developmental, transitional, and transformational change differ?
4 What are the key benefits and challenges when developing quality improvement programmes?

See the Appendix on page 254 for suggested answers to these questions.

References

Amarantou, V., Kazakopoulou, S., Chatzoudes, D. and Chatzoglou, P. (2018) Resistance to change: An empirical investigation of its antecedents, *Journal of Organisational Change Management*, 31 (2): 426–450.

Attree, M. (2007) Factors influencing nurses' decisions to raise concerns about care quality, *Journal of Nursing Management*, 15 (4): 392–402.

Auguste, J. (2013) Applying Kotter's 8-step process for leading change to the digital transformation of an orthopedic surgical practice group in Toronto, Canada, *Journal of Health Medical Information*, 4: 129. Available at: https://doi.org/10.4172/2157-7420.1000129.

Barr, J. and Dowding, L. (2012) *Leadership in Health Care*. London: Sage.

Barrett, G. (2003) How to manage change: The four A's of change, *Journal of Neonatal Nursing*, 9 (5): 153–157.

Beerel, A. (2009) *Leadership and Change Management*. London: Sage.

Bird, J. (2020) Using change management to implement barcode medicines administration technology, *Nursing Management*, 27 (5): 30–34.

Bishop, S. (2010) *Develop Your Assertiveness*. London: Kogan Page.

Broome, A. (1998) *Managing Change: Essentials of nursing management*, 2nd edition. London: Macmillan.

Brown, A. (2020) Communication and leadership in healthcare quality governance, *Journal of Health Organisational Management*, 34 (2): 144–162.

Bull, K. and Veall, A. (2009) Developing a diabetes link-nurse programme using the RAID quality improvement model, *Journal of Diabetes Nursing*, 13 (8): 298–304.

Burnes, B. (2004) Kurt Lewin and the planned approach to change: A re-appraisal, *Journal of Management Studies*, 4 (6): 977–1002.

Cahill, J. (1995) Innovation and the role of the change agent, *Professional Nurse*, 11 (1): 57–58.

Care Quality Commission (CQC) (2012) *The Speaking Up Charter.* Available at: https://www.cqc.org.uk/sites/default/files/documents/final_speaking_up_charter_cqc_version.pdf (accessed: 7 March 2021).

Care Quality Commission (CQC) (2018) *Opening the Door to Change: NHS safety culture and the need for transformation.* Available at: https://www.cqc.org.uk/publications/themed-work/opening-door-change (accessed: 25 June 2021).

Carnall, C. (2007) *Managing Change in Organisations.* Harlow: Prentice-Hall.

Chambers, R., Boath, E., and Rogers, D. (2007) *Clinical Effectiveness and Clinical Governance Made Easy*, 4th edition. Oxford: Radcliffe Publishing.

Chartered Society of Physiotherapy (CSP) (2019) *Code of Members' Professional Values and Behaviour.* Available at: https://www.csp.org.uk/publications/code-members-professional-values-behaviour (accessed: 7 March 2021).

Davies, A., James, W., and Griffiths, L. (2020) Implementing a quality improvement programme in a locality mental health service, *Nurse Management*, 27 (1): 27–32.

Department of Health (1998) *A First Class Service: Quality in the new NHS.* London: Department of Health.

Francis Report (2013) *Report of the Mid Staffordshire NHS Foundation Trust Public Inquiry.* London: HMSO.

Frawley, T., Meehan, A., and De Brun, A. (2018) Impact of organisational change for leaders in mental health, *Journal of Health Organisation and Management*, 32 (8): 980–1001.

Gillies, D.A. (1994) *Nursing Management: A systems approach*, 3rd edition. London: W.B. Saunders.

Graham, R.N.J. and Woodhead, T. (2021) Leadership for continuous improvement in healthcare during the time of COVID-19, *Clinical Radiology*, 76 (1): 67–72.

Health & Care Professions Council (HCPC) (2014) *Standards of Proficiency: Paramedics.* London: HCPC. Available at: https://www.hcpc-uk.org/resources/standards/standards-of-proficiency-paramedics/.

Heath, C. and Heath, D. (2013) *Switch: How to change things when change is hard.* London: Random House Business.

Hendry, C. (1996) Understanding and creating whole organizational change through learning theory, *Human Relations*, 48 (5): 621–641.

Hopson, B., Sacally, M. and Stafford, K. (2000) *Transitions: The challenge of change.* Chalford: Management Books.

Hospital Authority Hong Kong (2021) *Annual Report on Sentinel and Serious Untoward Events: October 2019–September 2020.* Available at: https://www.ha.org.hk/haho/ho/psrm/E_SESUE1920.pdf (accessed: 7 March 2021).

Iles, V. and Sutherland, K. (2001) *Organisational Change: A review for healthcare managers, professionals and researchers.* London: London School of Hygiene and Tropical Medicine.

Jackson, D., Peters, K., Andrew, S., Edenborough, M., Halcomb, E., Luck, L. *et al.* (2010) Understanding whistle-blowing: Qualitative insights from nurse whistle-blowers, *Journal of Advanced Nursing*, 66 (10): 2194–2201.

Jones, B., Vaux, E., and Olsson-Brown, A. (2019) How to get started in quality improvement, *British Medical Journal*, 364: k5408. Available at: https://doi.org/10.1136/bmj.k5437 (accessed: 7 March 2021).

Kenny, K., Vandekerckhove, W., and Fotaki, M. (2019) *The Whistleblowing Guide: Speak-up arrangements, challenges and best practice.* Chichester: Wiley.

Kotter, J. (2012) *Leading Change.* Boston, MA: Harvard Business Review Press.

Kotter, J. and Schlesinger, L. (2008) Choosing strategies for change, *Harvard Business Review*, July/August: 1–11. Available at: https://hbr.org/2008/07/choosing-strategies-for-change (accessed: 25 June 2021).

Kubler-Ross, E. (1969) *On Death and Dying.* New York: Macmillan.

Levine, K., Carmody, M., and Silk, K. (2020) The influence of organizational culture, climate and commitment on speaking up about medical errors, *Journal of Nursing Management*, 28 (1): 130–138.

Lewin, K. (1951) *Field Theory in Social Science.* New York: Harper & Row.

Lumbers, M. (2018) Approaches to leadership and managing change in the NHS, *British Journal of Nursing*, 27 (10): 554–558.

Marquis, B.L. and Huston, C.J. (1998) *Management Decision-making for Nurses: 124 case studies*, 3rd edition. Philadelphia, PA: Lippincott.

Maslow, A. (1954) *Motivation and Personality.* New York: Harper & Row.

McClelland, D. (1961) *The Achieving Society.* New York: Van Nostrand Reinhold.

McSherry, R. and Pearce, P. (2002) *Clinical Governance: A guide to implementation for healthcare professionals.* Oxford: Blackwell.

Mullins, L. (2010) *Management and Organisational Behaviour*, 9th edition. Harlow: Prentice-Hall.

NHS (2014) *Five Year Forward View.* Available at: https://www.england.nhs.uk/wp-content/uploads/2014/10/5yfv-web.pdf (accessed: 7 March 2012).

NHS (2019) *The NHS Long Term Plan.* Available at: https://www.longtermplan.nhs.uk/publication/nhs-long-term-plan/ (accessed: 7 March 2021).

NHS England (2017) *The Fifteen Steps Challenge. Quality from a patient's perspective: An inpatient toolkit.* Available at: https://www.england.nhs.uk/wp-content/uploads/2017/11/15-steps-inpatient.pdf (accessed: 24 March 2021)

NHS England and Health Education England (2018) *Leadership Development. Integrated urgent care / NHS 111 workforce blueprint.* Available at: https://www.england.nhs.uk/wp-content/uploads/2018/03/leadership-development.pdf (accessed: 25 June 2021).

NHS Leadership Academy (2013) *Developing Outstanding Leadership in Primary Care. What the NHS Leadership Academy can offer you.* Available at: https://www.leadershipacademy.nhs.uk (accessed: 7 March 2021).

Nilsen, P., Schildmeijer, K., Ericsson, C., Seingm, I., and Birken, S. (2019) Implementation of change in health care in Sweden: A qualitative study of professionals' change responses, *Implementation Science*, 14 (1): 51. Available at: https://doi.org/10.1186/s13012-019-0902-6 (accessed: 7 March 2021).

Nursing and Midwifery Council (NMC) (2015) *The Code: Professional standards of practice and behaviour for nurses, midwives and nursing associates.* London: NMC.

Parkin, P. (2009) *Managing Change in Healthcare: Using action research.* London: Sage.

Rogers, E. (1983) *Diffusion of Innovations.* New York: Free Press.

Rogers, P. (2006) RAID methodology: The NHS clinical governance team's approach to service improvement, *Clinical Governance: An International Journal*, 11 (1): 69–80.

Royal College of Occupational Therapists (RCOT) (2015) *Code of Ethics and Professional Conduct*, revised edition. Available at: https://www.rcot.co.uk/files/download-code-ethics-and-professional-conduct-occupational-therapists-2015 (accessed 25 June 2021).

Sale, D. (2005) *Understanding Clinical Governance and Quality Assurance: Making it happen.* Basingstoke: Palgrave Macmillan.

Sanchez-Cortes, D., Aran, O., Mast, M.S., and Gatica-Perez, D. (2012) A non-verbal behaviour approach to identify emergent leaders in small groups, *Multimedia*, 14 (3): 816–832.

Schwappach, D. and Gehring, K. (2014) Silence that can be dangerous: A vignette study to assess healthcare professionals' likelihood of speaking up about safety concerns, *PLoS One*, 9: e104720. Available at: https://doi.org/10.1371/journal.pone.0104720.

Seden, J., Matthews, S., McCormick, M. and Morgan, A. (2010) *Professional Development in Social Work*. London: Routledge.

Song, L., Park, B., and Oh, K.M. (2015) Analysis of the technology acceptance model in examining nurses' behavioral intention toward the use of barcode medication, *Computers, Informatics, Nursing*, 33 (4): 157–165.

Sullivan, E. and Garland, G. (2013) *Practical Leadership and Management in Healthcare: For nurses and allied health professionals*. London: Pearson.

Swage, T. (2004) *Clinical Governance in Healthcare Practice*. Oxford: Butterworth Heinemann.

Tannenbaum, R. and Schmidt, W.H. (1973) How to choose a leadership pattern, *Harvard Business Review*, 51 (3): 162–180.

The Health Foundation (2010) *Improvement in Practice: Beth Israel Deaconess case study. How leadership and a focus on quality rescued the Beth Israel Deaconess Medical Center*. London: The Health Foundation. Available at: https://www.health.org.uk/publications/case-study-beth-israel-deaconess-medical-center (accessed: 25 June 2021).

Veenstra, G.L., Ahaus, K., Welker, G.A., Heineman, E., van der Laan, M.J., and Muntinghe, F.L.H. (2017) Rethinking clinical governance. Healthcare professionals' views: A Delphi study, *BMJ Open*, 7: e012591. Available at: https://doi.org/10.1136/bmjopen-2016-012591.

Vroom, V.H. (1964) *Work and Motivation*. New York: Wiley.

Wu, S., Tyler, A., Logsdon, T., Holmes, N., Balkian, A., Brittan, M., La Vonda, H. *et al.* (2016) A quality improvement collaborative to improve the discharge process of hospitalized children, *Paediatrics*, 138 (2): e2014-3604. Available at: https://doi.org/10.1542/peds.2014-3604.

5 Implementing clinical governance strategies through education and training

Mary Gottwald

Learning objectives

By the end of this chapter, the reader will be better able to:

- Consolidate an understanding of lifelong learning and continuing professional development
- Understand how the TRAMm model can support you to engage with continuing professional development
- Identify a variety of methods that could be used to facilitate learning at all levels, through education and training

- Understand how education and training impact on the culture of organizations
- Understand how action learning sets can be used to facilitate continuing professional development

Introduction

The focus of this chapter is on education and training, which we believe to be one of the key strategies of clinical governance. Concepts of lifelong learning and continuing professional development will be explored as well as the need for cultural change within health and social care organizations. VARK will be introduced as a means to understanding one's own learning style, and practical suggestions on how education and training must be included at the individual, team, and organizational levels will be considered. The chapter will conclude with a discussion on organizational culture, by making links to education and training.

Clinical governance and continuing quality improvement (CQI) can only be successful if healthcare organizations value and empower their staff, both clinical and non-clinical, by having education and training structures in place. Two examples we provide illustrate where countries have recognized the importance of continuing professional development. Developing educational courses for healthcare professionals internationally is essential if safe and high-quality care is to be provided for service users.

Edwards (2018) highlights concerns regarding maternal mortality in Uganda. He states that most midwifery programmes delivered in Uganda are only of two years' duration and do not necessarily meet minimum standards from across the world. Therefore, there is a need to raise the level of midwifery education in order to improve the quality of care provided, and thus reduce maternal mortality and improve maternal and child health. There is also a need for Uganda to meet international Congress of Midwives Standards with mandatory post-registration professional development and regulation. However, Edwards suggests that other factors apart from the level of midwifery education have to be considered. For example, expectant mothers might delay seeking care, partly because they have so far to travel and then, once they do seek care, there may be a delay in the delivery of care. Edwards concludes that if midwifery education is developed and covers issues such as the above, midwives will have a better understanding of the factors that contribute to a delay in expectant mothers seeking support.

Nurakynova (2018), who conducted research into medical universities in Kazakhstan, takes this one step further by highlighting the need for all educational establishments delivering healthcare programmes to continuously improve educational governance, since this, in turn, will facilitate an improvement in the health and safety of patients. To demonstrate commitment to the development of medical courses so that they were more like those delivered across Europe and met international standards, Kazakhstan joined the Bologna Process in 2010. Launched in 1998–99, the Bologna Process established goals in participating countries for reform in higher education.

Learning

There is a plethora of literature in relation to learning, including the works of Bandura, Maslow, Piaget, Kolb, Dewey, Honey and Mumford, Skinner, and Pavlov. However, it is not the remit of this chapter to discuss these theorists, and readers with an interest should explore this literature independently.

Learning is a broad concept and involves changes in knowledge, skills, attitudes, and behaviour. It can be both formal and informal. In order to continuously update the evidence base of our practice and provide safe quality healthcare, learning must be lifelong and therefore ultimately this involves change (Mullins, 2010). Learning ought to be a feature of healthcare organizations, and strategies for staff development through continuing professional development should be a part of any organization's business plans (Gopee and Galloway, 2009).

There are many forms of learning:

Formal learning

Such learning takes place in the classroom, is assessed and qualifications may be awarded.

Informal learning

Learning can also be informal, opportunistic, and experiential, in that it occurs through observation within a social context and healthcare practice environment – in other words, learning whilst at work and learning from experiences that have occurred at work. An example of opportunistic learning is professional socialization (Brennan and McSherry, 2006; Jackson and Thurgate, 2011; Brown, Stevens, and Kermonde, 2013).

Professional socialization

Professional socialization can be defined as "a process whereby a person gains the knowledge, skills and identity that are characteristic of a professional and is a developmental process of adult socialization" (Becker Hentz, cited in Brown *et al.*, 2013: 555).

In their research, Brennan and McSherry (2006) explore the transitional process and professional socialization from healthcare assistant to student nurse. It can be extrapolated therefore that the same process will occur throughout pre-registration programmes. Healthcare students experience a transitional process whereby their behaviour changes in relation to their identity, occupational roles, and relationships, and consequently they become professionally socialized into their specific profession. This also involves assimilating the profession's values and norms, which are not necessarily teachable.

Professional socialization may include:

1 Culture shock
2 Anticipated socialization

Culture shock

Students may experience confusion in relation to understanding their occupational role identity, which could lead to role conflict and role ambiguity, and hence some students may take longer to socialize into their profession (Brown *et al.*, 2013). Brennan and McSherry (2006) identify this confusion as experiencing a culture shock. Not only do students have to learn about the theory underpinning practice but also about professional aspects such as accountability, professional responsibility, and professional and ethical codes of conduct. Culture shock may become transition shock as students enter their first role as a newly graduated nurse and need to immerse themselves into potentially stressful and intense professional practice (Duchscher, 2009).

Anticipated socialization

Prior work experience whilst at school may have included working in a nursing home or rehabilitation ward, and as a result of this experience students may enter their pre-registration programme with ideas about the values of their profession and have a comfortable feeling when working within healthcare. Brown *et al.* (2013: 565) suggest the term "anticipated socialization".

However, pre-registration placements could include working in other more challenging areas such as psychiatric units, prisons, or specialized burns units, and so students will need to go through a transitional period adapting and developing their knowledge and skills to enable them to work in these varied areas of practice, some of which could be challenging. Pre-registration students who have undertaken prior work experience will have gained knowledge as well as practical experience and consequently could be considered to be at an advantage. However, transferring this to different settings and adapting may take time, therefore professional socialization can be challenging for everyone.

Lifelong learning

On graduation, pre-registration students are deemed to have achieved professional socialization. However, this should not be the end of their learning journey, and, as already stated, lifelong learning is imperative if organizations are to constantly improve the quality of healthcare provision. "Lifelong learning depends on every health organisation developing its learning environment" (Swage, 2004: 180) into one that is conducive to learning. Lifelong learning involves "changes and learning that continue throughout life, and takes places in a variety of ways and range of situations" (Mullins, 2010: 172).

It is therefore vital that healthcare organizations become learning organizations. This will be discussed in more detail towards the end of this chapter iwhen we address organizational culture.

Continuing professional development

Lifelong learning includes continuing professional development (CPD). The Heath and Care Professions Council (HCPC, 2018) define CPD as "the way in which registrants continue to learn and develop throughout their careers so they keep their skills and knowledge up to date and are able to practise safely and effectively".

HCPC (2018) state that all health and social care professionals must meet five CPD standards.

Activity 5.1

Access the following link and reflect on the five CPD standards:

https://www.hcpc-uk.org/cpd/your-cpd/our-standards-for cpd/ (accessed: 7 March 2021)

Reflect on your practice over the last week and consider examples that demonstrate where you have met these standards.

As part of continuing registration, CPD is mandatory in the UK for all healthcare professionals and should commence as soon as individuals have qualified and are registered to practise. Hearle, Lawson, and Morris (2016) suggest that CPD should be part of all healthcare professionals' contracts, including administrative, domestic, and technical staff. In the European Union (EU), "CPD is an ethical obligation for all health professionals to ensure their professional practice is up-to-date and can contribute to improving patient outcomes and quality of care" (EAHC, 2013: 6). Even though there is disparity in the requirements across the EU, there is no evidence to suggest that one country's approach to CPD is superior to that of another.

Further afield, registered nurses in Hong Kong are also required to undertake CPD. In any three-year period, it is mandatory for a registered nurse to gain 45 continuing nurse education points (CNE) and an enrolled nurse 35 CNE points. One point is equivalent to one hour of learning.

It is clear that CPD should be mandatory for all healthcare professionals across the world. Should you be planning to develop your experience in another country, it is essential that you check what CPD is required.

Table 5.1 considers a number of CPD definitions other than that of the HCPC (2018) above, and identifies some strengths and limitations. One of the advantages of the definitions proposed by Wright and Hill (2003) and Swage (2004) is that the focus is on both the individual and the organization. Education and training related to the individual and organizational levels will be considered later in the chapter.

Figure 5.1, which is discussed later in the chapter, exemplifies how the aims of CPD can be illustrated by a continuous cycle of events. It also depicts how CPD is linked with appraisal.

Table 5.1 Definitions of continuing professional development

Definition	Critique
Wright and Hill (2003: 85) "A purposeful, systematic activity by individuals and possibly their organisations, to maintain and develop the knowledge, skills and attributes which are needed for effective professional practice"	Includes both the individual and organization Focus is wider than just knowledge
Swage (2004: 6) CPD programmes are "aimed at meeting the development needs of individual health professionals, and the service needs of the organisation are in place and supported locally and regularly monitored"	Includes both the individual and organization Focus is on regular evaluation
Mullins (2010: 824) "The process of planned, continuing development of individuals throughout their career"	Does not consider the needs of the organization
Swage (2004: 318) "An individual taking responsibility for the development of his/her own career by systematically analysing development needs, identifying and using appropriate methods to meet these needs and regularly reviewing achievement compared against personal and career objectives"	Does not consider the needs of the organization Focus is on regular review and monitoring of objectives

Figure 5.1 CPD cycle

| Assessment of individual's needs |
| Assessment of organization's needs |

| Evaluation of the CPD process |
| Evaluation of benefits to the individual, patient, and organization |

| Agreement of Personal Development Plans (PDP) / Personal Development Reviews (PDR) with ALL staff |

| Identification of training and education needs |
| Implementation of agreed objectives |

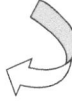

Adapted from: Sale (2005: 96).

Aims of continuing professional development

There are two key aims of CPD (Swage, 2004):

1 To ensure that healthcare professionals are provided with opportunities to develop their attributes, knowledge, and skills so they are enabled to progress along their career pathway. This impacts on the second aim:
2 To ensure services continue to develop and provide an improved patient experience

Self-development, therefore, is very much part of CPD, and keeping a portfolio and undertaking a minimum number of hours' learning is a requirement of many healthcare professions if individuals wish to retain their registration. The reason is that practitioners need to demonstrate that they are continually learning and updating their practice. However, in their research with nurses and allied health professionals, Haywood *et al.* (2013) identified insufficient time and lack of funding as two of the key barriers to healthcare professionals undertaking CPD. If there is an expectation that staff will contribute to, if not pay for all of, their CPD, as well as carry out their CPD activities in their own time, it is likely to impact on whether they engage with more than the basic requirements (Haywood *et al.*, 2013). In addition, healthcare professionals in developing nations may well not be in a position to either access or pay for CPD in their own time. Haywood *et al.* also highlight that engaging with CPD becomes demotivating if staff find it difficult to apply their CPD learning to practice and/or if it does not lead to career progression. Due to funding limitations within healthcare organizations, as discussed earlier in this chapter, there is perhaps a greater need to engage in informal experiential learning. Haywood *et al.* suggest that recruiting experienced staff within an organization to deliver CPD would be more cost-effective, although such in-house learning might not be delivered in sufficient depth.

Hearle *et al.* (2016) suggest the TRAMm circular model framework is a useful way to ensure health and social care professionals undertake CPD activities. This model can be used by individuals or organizations to guide staff members in their CPD development, thus moving the organization to a culture of learning.

There are five core aspects of this model:

1 Tell
2 Record
3 Activity
4 Monitor
5 Measure

This model uses an outcomes-based approach to help individuals reflect on their practice. Using these five core aspects to guide them can help health and social care professionals to meet the five HCPC standards (HCPC, 2018). Individuals need to consider gaps in their knowledge, plan their future learning, consider how they will apply their learning to practice, and lastly, and perhaps most importantly, how they will evaluate what impact their CPD activities will have on future patient care. In other words, it is not good enough just to attend CPD courses. Acquiring and applying this new learning adds to values-based practice discussed in Chapter 6.

Activity 5.2

You may find the following links useful when considering the TRAMm model:

https://trammcpd.com/ (accessed: 7 March 2021)
https://trammcpd.com/free-downloads (accessed: 7 March 2021)

Action learning and continuing professional development

James and Stacey-Emile (2019) discuss how action learning is a useful way for nurses and midwives to engage with CPD through a problem-solving approach and therefore meet all requirements for nursing bodies. Gillett, Reed, and Bryan (2017) add that action learning sets are useful for all healthcare professionals. Action learning "is an approach to problem solving and learning in groups to bring about change in individuals, teams, organisations and systems" (Pedlar, 2008: 1), and therefore an essential feature of a learning organization engaged in bringing about a change in practice as discussed later in this chapter. Action learning involves healthcare professionals volunteering to join an action learning set and being prepared to work in small groups of six to eight individuals. Each group requires a facilitator who will initially need to explain the aim and address the ground rules, confidentiality, etc. (James and Stacey-Emile, 2019). It is also essential that the members of the learning set have support from management (Gillett *et al.*, 2017); if not, this might impact on whether action plans are implemented successfully.

There is an expectation that members of the set will be committed and that they will also learn from this experience, which is learn by doing, so has some similarities to quality circles discussed in Chapter 1. Action learning sets are empowering and allow time for staff to reflect, share, and discuss their experiences, whilst also learning from other members of the group and developing their own knowledge. Members of the learning set must be prepared to challenge (not in a confrontational manner) others and be challenged themselves. An important aspect of action learning sets is for the discussions to culminate in agreed action plans and, as with all action plans, there needs to be an evaluation to identify if change has taken place (James and Stacey-Emile, 2019).

Individuals can take responsibility and can bring current quality issues, near miss incidences, or any concerns with the safety of patients to the group. Taking responsibility sits with the definitions of clinical governance offered in Chapter 1. For example, following the CQC review of mental health services (2014–2017) outlined in Chapter 1, staff working within mental health services may decide to set up an action learning set to help them to further engage with CPD to facilitate change and thereby lead to improved quality healthcare provision.

Gillett *et al.* (2017) provide an example of how action learning sets can be used to support and improve end-of-life care. The Quality End-of-life Care for All (QELCA) programme was initially established by a hospice in London, although the five-day programme is now delivered to multidisciplinary teams in a variety of healthcare settings. On alternate days of the programme, participants attend the hospice as usual, which is important as it gives them time to apply their learning to practice and embraces the learn-by-doing theme mentioned above. Those attending the programme need to be in senior positions within their hospices, so that they can facilitate change with the support of management. Management is also asked to agree and give support to the action plans. Specialists from the hospice are also part of the discussions so that they can ensure individual action plans are credible and pragmatic.

Following the five-day programme, participants join an action learning set which meets monthly for a period of six months in the participants' workplace and continues to be supported by the same facilitator who delivered the initial programme. If possible, a hospice specialist also joins the action learning set so they can keep abreast of ideas and support staff to undertake and apply these ideas in practice. "The action learning sets focus on leading and managing change for 'self' and the 'team' and on effectively overcoming obstacles to the delivery of acceptable end-of-life care in practice" (Gillett *et al.*, 2017: 188). It is important to note that each member of the group is given equal time to present concerns and propose ideas and action plans and the other members are given time to seek clarification and make recommendations. It is the facilitator's responsibility to ensure the process for an action learning set is followed and then to summarize and keep a note of the future actions to be undertaken. At the beginning of the next meeting, each member of the learning set will share the impact of their action plan (Haith, 2012)

As with any new initiative or change to practice, the QELCA programme did face challenges. However, it is evident from interviews undertaken as part of the evaluation of the programme and learning sets, that the programme does work for individuals and teams and that it has a positive impact on the quality of end-of-life care for both patients and their families (Gillett *et al.*, 2017). This programme also demonstrates that working as a team/small group can be more influential and effective than working alone.

James and Stacey-Emile (2019) state that managers must be prepared to allocate time for action learning sets and must also be prepared to allocate resources for the development of staff skills. This can be seen as a potential challenge to the success of action learning sets. Action learning sets also help individuals to develop their own skills, including their communication skills, leadership skills, problem-solving skills (e.g. why an action taken worked or did not work), critical analytical skills, presentation skills, analytical and reflective skills – such as when considering action plans. Other skills include planning, listening, challenging, working as a team, and being willing to support others. Lastly, similar to quality circles, action learning sets allow individuals to be creative with ideas (Pedlar, 2008; Gillett *et al.*, 2017; James and Stacey-Emile, 2019).

Individual, team, and organizational levels of education and training

In order to improve the quality of care provided and to guarantee standards are met, clinicians need to ensure that they have up-to-date skills and knowledge and, as discussed in Chapters 1 and 7, must make sure their practice is evidence-based. Links to clinical governance therefore need to be made between clinical effectiveness, research, and development of practice. Organizations have to make certain that staff employed have the right attributes as well as skills and knowledge. However, responsibility does not solely lie with the organization, and Sale (2005) suggests that education and training should occur at three levels: individual, team, and organization. Figure 5.2 illustrates some educational activities that can be carried out at each of these levels.

Figure 5.2 Levels of education and training

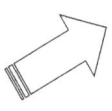

INDIVIDUAL LEVEL

- Engage in short courses, e-learning, distance learning (Massive Online Open Courses), postgraduate courses
- Reflective diaries
- Use time outside of work

TEAM LEVEL

- Multidisciplinary teams
- Workshops
- Seminars/lectures/tutorials
- Critical incidents
- Case studies
- Journal clubs
- Simulations

EDUCATION AND TRAINING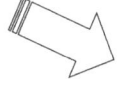

ORGANIZATIONAL LEVEL

- Induction/preceptorship programmes
- Provision of resources
- Provision of mandatory training

Adapted from: Wright and Hill (2003), Sale (2005).

Individual level

As discussed in Chapter 1, practitioners are accountable and therefore responsible for making sure their practice is evidence-based. This also links to effectiveness, one of Maxwell's six dimensions of quality discussed in Chapter 3. However, finances within health and social care organizations are limited and therefore individuals may need to use some of their personal time as well as finances outside work to develop their knowledge.

Individuals must make sure they engage with and complete all mandatory training and they could also utilize opportunities to engage in e-learning/online distance learning/Massive Online Open Courses (MOOCs), short courses (both accredited and non-accredited), postgraduate certificates, diplomas, or Masters programmes. They could access the organization's Learning and Development Centre to identify relevant training opportunities delivered within the organization.

Individuals could also undertake a SWOT analysis as discussed in Chapter 3. Having reflected on their strengths, weakness, opportunities, and threats, further learning can be facilitated through setting mutually agreed objectives and action plans linked to the SWOT analysis. These objectives need to be agreed with their line manager. Individuals need to engage with agreed objectives and review these objectives at their next annual personal development review (or appraisal). It is also useful to have an interim review to check progress and to see if further support is needed from line managers so that action plans are fulfilled (Wright and Hill, 2003; Sale, 2005).

Activity 5.3

In 2012, the Department of Health published *Liberating the NHS: Developing the Healthcare Workforce. From Design to Delivery*. The Education Outcomes Framework (EOF) included in this document aims to make sure that staff "have the right skills, behaviours and training, available in the right numbers, to support the delivery of excellent healthcare and health improvement" (2013: 4). The EOF can be seen to be a facilitator of improvement in the quality and safety of patient health and social care. For a wider understanding on Department of Health plans, access The Education Outcomes Framework (2013) at the following link:

https://assets.publishing.service.gov.uk/government/uploads/system/uploads/attachment_data/file/175546/Education_outcomes_framework.pdf (accessed: 7 March 2021)

It is also important if you work within the UK to make sure you are familiar with the NHS Knowledge and Skills Framework. In 2019, this was simplified to cover six core dimensions required for all jobs. For further reading, access:

https://www.nhsemployers.org/SimplifiedKSF (accessed: 7 March 2021)

Consider your own area of practice.

- What recent education and training have you undertaken at the individual level?
- Are you using the TRAMm model framework to guide your reflections, to monitor and evaluate your learning?

Identifying individual learning needs

There are a number of methods that are used to identify individual learning needs. This chapter will consider VARK.

VARK

VARK is a short questionnaire devised by Fleming in 1987. It is accessible in a variety of languages and is quick to complete online as it only contains 16 questions. Fleming stresses that VARK is not a learning style inventory as such because it looks at one aspect only. It does not consider dimensions such as when individuals like to learn or what motivates them to engage in small group work or one-to-one tutorials, for example. Despite this, it is still useful and can be used by individuals to help them further understand how they learn best.

It could also be used within teams to help understand individual differences and build relationships. When using VARK, all copyright regulations must be adhered to.

Activity 5.4

- Access the VARK website and complete the questionnaire: http://www.vark-learn.com/english
- Once you have identified your preference(s), access the help sheets, which will provide strategies to facilitate your learning.

Once you have completed the VARK questionnaire, you will have identified your learning preferences and these are shown in Table 5.2.

We have considered a variety of methods that could be used to facilitate learning at the individual level. The next activity will help you to link your learning preferences to methods of learning.

Activity 5.5

- Having identified your learning preferences, consider which methods suit you best.
- Do practical simulations and workshops, lectures, online learning opportunities, case study or journal club discussions suit your learning preferences?
- Which of the strategies identified in VARK could facilitate your learning further?

Table 5.2 Dimensions of VARK

Visual	Individuals with this preference like to learn from graphs, mind maps, histograms, etc. – that is, any symbolic or graphic form
Auditory	Listening to oral presentations is preferred and these individuals also like to engage and interact with lectures, seminars, and discussion groups
Read/write	Diaries, lists, bullet points, handouts, and leaflets are preferred methods of learning
Kinaesthetic	Here learning takes place through all senses and these individuals like to learn through concrete examples and in particular like to be able to link these examples to their own experience

Linking learning needs and personal development reviews

The flow diagram in Figure 5.3 illustrates four steps that could help you to prepare for your next personal development review (PDR) and development of your personal development plan (PDP).

Writing objectives

When writing objectives, they need to be SMART (Mullins, 2010):

- Specific
- Measurable
- Achievable
- Realistic/relevant
- Timeframe/time-bound

If each objective contains all of the above elements, it is much easier to evaluate and measure. For example:

1 By the end of 2022, I will submit an article to a peer-reviewed journal
2 By the end of July 2022, I will have read at least one journal article per month

---

Activity 5.6

Consider the above writing objectives.

- Are they SMART? If so, why? If not, why not?
- Does your team set SMART objectives?

Team level

Education and training at this level probably works best if delivered to multidisciplinary teams, as this fosters better communication and collaboration and understanding of roles. One advantage of learning in teams is that members tend to have the shared value "to meet the needs of their patients" (Wright and Hill, 2003: 168). Further education and training may be one of the requirements following a near miss event or a complaint, to ensure that the mistake does not happen again.

As has been discussed previously, near miss events are events that should and can be avoided. Vásquez-Sánchez et al. (2020) carried out a small study within a primary healthcare setting in Spain to understand what near misses

Figure 5.3 Identifying learning development

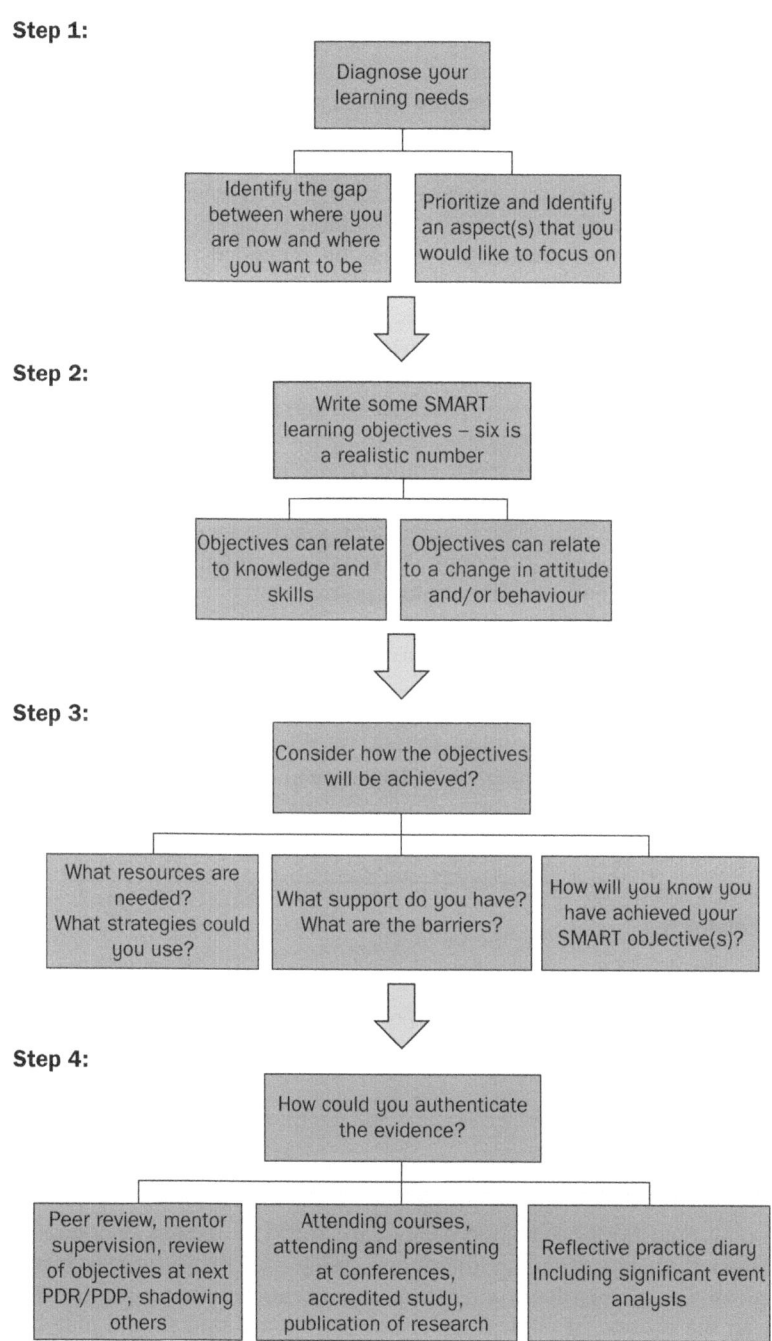

Adapted from: Swage (2004: 181).

occurred and the reasons for them. Four experienced nurses completed a questionnaire on near miss events. They identified that 185 near miss events occurred in 2018 within primary healthcare, including an incorrect dose of medication, wrong concentration of medication, no record kept of patient allergies, and poor hand hygiene. Vásquez-Sánchez *et al.* (2020) concluded that most near misses were the result of administration or communication errors. Pressures of work, poor communication between doctors and nurses, and a fear of speaking up were cited as the causes of these near misses. Thus, education and training are key, and managers must be mindful of the need to allow teams time to continue their learning. Staff need to be reminded of the importance of reporting and recording near miss events. However, managers also have responsibilities, such as ensuring that staff feel confident about reporting an event and that blame will not be unfairly apportioned. An understanding of risk management within education and training sessions would also facilitate learning with regards to improving patient safety and avoiding near misses.

A variety of methods could be used to facilitate learning at the team level. For example, small group work could be organized, in which case studies and/or critical incidents are discussed and action plans agreed. Journal clubs could be established, in which all members agree to read and discuss one paper per month in small groups. Alternatively, members could take it in turns to agree to read and present key points from a current journal article, which may help to reduce time pressures. Workshops could be organized using manikins, and actors could be employed to role-play scenarios as a precursor to discussion.

All of the above encourage reflective practice and facilitate understanding of current practice and the evidence base for this. Learning can also be shared in everyday practice through peer observation and demonstration and through mentoring undergraduates, new graduates, and healthcare assistants (Sale, 2005).

Activity 5.7

Consider your own area of practice.

- What education and training are provided at the team level?
- Have you been provided with recent opportunities to engage in further learning at the team level?

Organizational level

From the outset, all health and social care staff can expect structures to be provided that include induction/preceptorship and mentoring programmes. They can also expect the organization to provide continuous clinical supervision. In the context of clinical governance, the induction should also include learning activities so that staff can understand the clinical governance framework, how this framework links to the organization's strategic directives as well as government directives, and their role in ensuring clinical governance strategies are implemented. In order for education and training to be successful, the organization must provide resources, both in terms of finances and time, so that development objectives identified in personal development plans can be achieved. Resources also need to be provided to enable mandatory training to be completed, for example health and safety, infection and prevention procedures, moving and handling, resuscitation. Nowadays, some of this mandatory training takes place through e-learning.

One of the advantages of e-learning is that staff can learn at a time that suits them. However, organizations must still allow dedicated time for this learning and staff need to manage their time to ensure this learning takes place. E-learning may include online learning that organizations have developed and so is accessible only to employees of that organization, or courses provided by universities that are open only to those registered on specific programmes. E-learning may also include courses known as MOOCs. Since 2007, there has been a move for institutions to provide opportunities for learners to engage in Massive Open Online Courses (MOOCs). MOOCs originated in Canada and up to a point are free of charge. They provide opportunities for those interested in learning to engage in flexible, open access, non-credited courses accessed via the web. Anyone throughout the world with a desire to develop their learning can register. Although non-credited, assessments are included and on successful completion of the course, certificates are provided. One of the advantages of MOOCs is that individuals can liaise across the world, sharing ideas and experiences (Daniel, 2012).

Activity 5.8

Consider your own area of practice.

- What education and training are provided at the organizational level?
- Have you been provided with recent opportunities to engage in further learning at the organizational level?

Learning organizations

We have discussed the importance of learning at the individual, team, and organizational levels. An organization in which learning is fostered is known as a learning organization. This type of organization continually provides opportunities for employees to develop their knowledge and skills in order to provide excellent quality care. A learning organization is one that "encourages and facilitates the learning and development of people at all levels of the organisation, values the learning and simultaneously transforms itself" (Mullins, 2010: 827), so that it become "an efficient adaptive unit" (Wright and Hill, 2003: 193).

Characteristics of a learning organization

There are a number of characteristics that identify whether an organization is a learning organization or not (Reineck, 2002; Mullins, 2010; Barr and Dowding, 2012):

- Staff feel that what they do is important and valued (see Schein's (2010) middle level of organizational culture, values, and beliefs, discussed below). If staff feel valued and therefore more motivated, staff retention will be high
- Staff are continually provided with opportunities to develop their knowledge and skills in relation to patient care. They are encouraged to try different approaches. They are also encouraged and facilitated to gain an understanding of how the different levels of the organization function
- Staff are encouraged to evaluate interventions and explore the strengths and limitations of these interventions
- There is mutual respect amongst employees and staff as different grades work together as colleagues, supporting each other in their learning (see Schein's (2010) inner layer of organizational culture underlying assumptions, discussed below)
- There is a shared vision within teams
- Communication is good at all levels

Activity 5.9

Reflect on the examples of poor quality care given in Chapter 1 (Figures 1.1 and 1.2). Do you think these were learning organizations? If not, why not?

Gopee and Galloway (2009) suggest that a positive organizational culture can impact on the likelihood of that organization becoming a learning organization.

Organizational culture

For staff to be able to engage in lifelong learning and CPD, the organizational culture needs to support learning. Culture is "something that is shared by members of an organisation ... the glue that holds together potentially diverse individuals" (Kelemen, 2005: 128). Mullins defines it as "how things are done around here" (2010: 739); in other words, what behaviour is acceptable and what behaviour is unacceptable. Huczynski and Buchanan provide us with a more in-depth definition: "Culture is the collection of relatively uniform and enduring values, beliefs, customs, traditions and practices that are shared by an organisation's members, learned by new recruits, and transmitted from one generation of employees to the next" (2007: 623).

This definition closely links to Schein's (2010) levels of culture, which will be discussed below. Clinical governance is about changing organizational culture in a systematic and demonstrable way, moving away from a culture of blame to one of learning, so that quality infuses all aspects of the organization's work (Department of Health, 1998). However, it is important to remember that organizational culture is not tangible and is hard to measure (Carnall, 2007).

Models of organizational culture

There are a number of models of organizational culture, such as those of Schein (2010) and Handy (1999), Johnson's (1988) cultural web, and Hofstede's (1968) characteristics of culture. Those of Schein (2010) and Handy (1999) will be discussed in more detail.

Levels of organizational culture

If staff accept the traditions, values, and beliefs held within the organization, they are more likely to become motivated and inspired to learn, and therefore the organization's strategic objectives are more likely to be achieved.

Schein (2010) identifies three levels of organizational culture, which can be depicted by the three layers of an onion (Figure 5.4).

1 Artefacts
2 Values and beliefs
3 Underlying assumptions

Figure 5.4 Layers of organizational culture

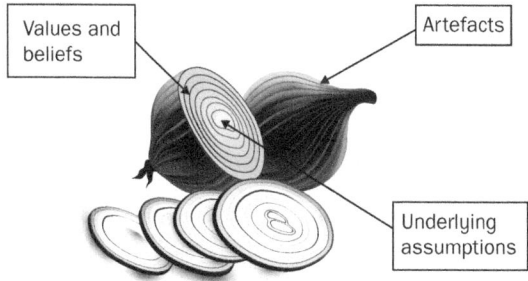

Artefacts

This is the outer and most superficial layer of the onion. Schein (2010) states that artefacts within the organization are tangible. They can be seen by everyone whether employed or not, for example:

* Furniture: the type of office furniture reflects certain privileges and grades
* Equipment
* Logos used on headed notepaper, or on signs at entrances to hospitals or community centres
* Uniforms that identify different staff (porters, nurses, doctors, allied health professionals, canteen staff)

Artefacts can also be heard and experienced, and include the behaviours that staff follow such as how staff speak to one another and display their emotions. In some organizations, this could be a bullying and blame culture, as discussed in Chapter 2. If the culture within the organization is one of bullying and blame, this could impede learning. Artefacts also include other behavioural manifestations such as rituals, for example the hospital ward round.

Values and beliefs

These form the middle layer of the onion and are not visible. Schein (2010) further suggests that individuals have their own notions on what is right and wrong. Organizational culture at this level will occur once the team agree and adopt shared beliefs, such as the importance of providing quality healthcare or reporting adverse incidents, for example needle stick or medication errors.

This layer includes unwritten rules (norms) that inform employees how to behave in a wide variety of situations. For example, not all health and social care professionals wear uniforms, in particular in the community and in mental health organizations, yet there is an expectation that staff and students on placement will present themselves in a professional manner. If the beliefs and values of a team are different from those that support high performance, the desired behaviour will not be reflected in the observed behaviour. Norms and values are linked. The norm of not displaying emotion whilst at work is linked to the value of self-discipline. Members of an organization that has a specific culture will hold values and conform to cultural norms, because their underlying assumptions support these values and norms.

Underlying assumptions

Underlying assumptions are at the deepest level, form the centre of the onion, and are not visible. Schein (2010) suggests that these underlying assumptions form the core of an organization's culture. There may be an underlying assumption that experienced senior staff are respected and so students on clinical placement become socialized to accept the cultural value of respecting senior staff. When a solution to a problem is found to be successful, then the method is repeated. These then become unconscious behaviours that are accepted and taken for granted.

When staff work towards continuous quality improvement (CQI), there is a quality culture within the organization. Strong organizational cultures work towards achieving common goals and standards (total quality management – TQM), and reward and value staff, who in turn are more likely to become motivated and inspired to engage in lifelong learning and CPD activities. Chapter 6 will discuss these concepts in greater detail.

Cultural types

Handy (1999) considers four types of culture that can exist within an organization:

1 Power culture
2 Role culture
3 Task culture
4 Person culture

Each cultural type has its strengths and limitations, some of which are identified in Table 5.3.

Power culture

This can be depicted as a spider's web where centralized control is undertaken by one individual or a few key individuals. There are "rays of power and influence [that spread] out from the central figure" (Handy, 1999: 184) and the closer individuals are to the centre, the greater their influence and power.

Role culture

Handy (1999) depicts this culture as a Greek temple. The pillars of this temple are independent departments such as the Human Resource Department, Learning and Development Centre, Finance Department, Physiotherapy Department, and Accident and Emergency Department. These departments support the pediment at the top of the temple. Within each department staff are employed because they have the skills and attributes required for the job. Staff are given a contract which includes a job description that identifies their key roles and responsibilities. The pediment of this temple can be seen as the senior management who are responsible for coordinating all procedures.

Table 5.3 Critique of cultural types

	Strengths	Limitations
Power	Will respond quickly to incidents Decisions are taken on the balance of influence Decisions made by a few individuals	Dependent on the capabilities of the key individuals at the centre Continued success may depend on succession
Role	Formal departments coordinated by senior management Standardization occurs through common procedures Rewards staff through promotion	Due to the formality of role culture, organizations may be slow to recognize the need to change and are slow to undertake change Individuals who are accustomed to power can become disillusioned
Task	Jobs and projects get completed by empowered teams The right individuals are employed with the right knowledge and skills	Relies on good collaboration and teamwork Individuals may lack the skills that role cultures possess Individual needs are less important than team needs
Person	The individual is the focal point and their basic needs are adhered to	Minimalistic structure The organization is subservient to the individual where individuals do their own thing

Adapted from: Handy (1999).

Rewards tend to occur within this culture. Opportunities are provided for further staff development through education and training, and this can lead to promotion within the organization. However, there are occasions when teams will come together to work on a specific task. In such cases, there may be conflicts over leadership of the newly formed group and the security of role culture may be undermined.

Task culture

"Task culture is job or project orientated" (Handy, 1999: 187) and can be depicted as a grid with the power lying at the junctures. The focus of this culture is to ensure the job or project is completed and therefore the right people with the right skills are employed and are accountable for particular jobs or projects. Organizations must ensure that these individuals are provided with further CPD opportunities. Individuals identify with the strategic objectives or the organization and work together so that the job is completed.

Person culture

Handy (1999) depicts this culture as a constellation of stars. It is unlikely that this culture is found solely in health and social care organizations, because person culture lacks structure and corporate objectives. As the structure is minimal, individuals are enabled to do their own thing more effectively.

Activity 5.10

Consider your own organization.

- Is there a predominant culture or is there a mix of cultures within your organization?
- Where does it fit in with Handy's (1999) descriptions of organizational culture (power, role, task, or person culture)?
- Is the emphasis on getting the job done (task culture)?
- Do the demands come from the top without much concern for your welfare as a person (power culture)?
- Are employees involved in decision-making (role culture)?
- Are there support mechanisms for staff, for example to manage stress within the working environment (person culture)?
- How do you as an individual relate to the culture in your organization?

Reflect on these questions and consider the rationale that supports your answers.

Worked examples of education and training

This book has considered a number of quality issues – pressure ulcers, medication errors, falls, ventilator-associated pneumonia, needle stick and sharps injuries, hospital-acquired infections, as well as violence, bullying, and aggression. Tables 5.4 to 5.10 identify some examples of education and training at each of the levels discussed above.

All of the methods mentioned have their strengths and limitations and therefore learners need to think about their learning styles, as this will help identify methods that most suit their needs. Table 5.11 begins to identify strengths and limitations. However, what has not been included in this table is the requirement to be aware of learners' individual learning preferences.

Table 5.4   Pressure ulcers

Individual level
* Ensure awareness of wound management policy and how to report near misses

Team level
* Mandatory training on venous thrombotic embolisms to ensure pressure ulcers do not occur due to immobilization
* Education and training needs assessment of teams. If staff make an error due to lack of awareness, then education and training must be provided, for example lack of awareness of who is at risk of developing a pressure sore due to poor nutrition, and the importance of hydration in relation to pressure sores
* Regular audits will lead to education and training if the incidence of pressure ulcers increases. For example, ensuring staff know the specialist beds that should be used or the requirements to regularly turn and examine common areas of risk
* Increase staff awareness on operational processes to be followed

Organizational level
* The incidence of pressure ulcers is auditable and therefore teams need to be aware of this
* Ensure staff are aware of NICE guidelines (http://nice.org.uk) and European guidelines, for example: http://epuap.org/guidelines (pressure ulcers)

Table 5.5   Medication errors

Individual level
* Ensure awareness of own professional responsibility and subsequent development in the safe administration of medications
* Ensure awareness of the trust policy on report medication errors

Team level
* Following a near miss or medication error, CPD is important to ensure that double checking or three checks and five rights (right drug to the right patient in the right dose by the right route at the right time) procedures are followed (ISMP, 2007)
* Workshop following a near miss – use this as a learning opportunity for the team, so that it is not the last domino who gets the blame

Organizational level
* During induction, all staff will be made aware of the procedural rules designed by the organization to follow the five rights. Organizations may consider adding three further rights (right reason, right drug formulation, and right line attachment) (ISMP, 2007)

Table 5.6 Falls

Individual level
- Regardless of lack of time, staff must remind each other to make sure the cot sides are put back up when required (for example, patient may have post-surgery psychosis or mental health issues)

Team level
- Supporting the education of teams in the use of risk assessment tools, for example the Morse Falls Risk Assessment
- Ensure staff are aware of the falls team and how to contact this team
- Remind staff of processes to follow after an incident or near miss

Organizational level
- Dissemination of communication guidelines to all staff, to raise awareness of local processes

Table 5.7 Ventilator-associated pneumonia

Individual level
- Ensure awareness of own professional development by being up to date on the management of ventilated patients and risks associated with the development of complications from mechanical ventilation, including VAP

Team level
- Increasing staff awareness of the availability of care bundles. See NICE guidelines for further details: http://www.NICE.org.UK/guidance/index.jsp?action=articleando=38047

Organizational level:
- During induction, all staff will be made aware of policies and procedures in place in ICUs, high-dependency units, and specialized wards to support withdrawal from mechanical ventilation and thereby a reduction in VAP
- Staff will also need to be made aware of the policies on how to reduce the risk once extubated on the high-dependency unit, ICU, or specialized unit

Table 5.8 Needle stick and sharps injuries

Individual level
- Own personal and professional responsibility to ensure up to date on needle stick and sharps injury policy, including how to avoid and so minimize the risk and how to report and what action is required if a needle stick injury occurs

Team level
- Ward information provided on location of sharps bins

(Continues)

Table 5.8 (Continued)

- Best practice would include regular training on the processes to follow in order to prevent needle stick injuries
- Processes accessible so that if a needle stick injury happens, staff know what process to follow

Organizational level
- Supported by the Occupational Health Department
- During induction, all staff will be made aware of processes and procedures in place to support the prevention of injuries, reporting of near misses or actual injuries

Table 5.9 Violence, bullying, and aggression

Individual level
- Organizational policy varies and therefore staff must ensure they are aware of local policy. They also need to check to see if it includes policies to follow for both verbal intimidation and physical aggression

Team level
- Team updates on current prevention and management of violence, bullying, and aggression
- Practice in breakaway techniques
- Make sure staff are aware of how to access procedural documents

Organizational level
- Mandatory training – prevention and management of violence, bullying, and aggression programmes, as well as breakaway techniques

Table 5.10 Hospital-acquired infections

Individual level
- Own personal and professional responsibility to ensure up to date on needle stick and sharps injury policy, including how to avoid and so minimize the risk and how to report and what action is required if an injury occurs
- Undertake mandatory training in hand washing, non-touch technique (NTT), *Clostridium difficile*, and MRSA

Team level
- Infection and prevention control nurse will provide regular updates on incidence of HAIs within the organization and therefore support training, for example isolation management

Organizational level
- Induction programmes to make staff aware of local policies and audit processes

---

Activity 5.11

Whilst you can engage in formal CPD events at the three levels discussed above, personal reading still remains key to personal development. The following will provide you with further information on the quality issues discussed in Chapter 2:

- The *Wound Repair and Regeneration* journal and *American Journal of Critical Care* (pressure ulcers)
- The *Journal of the American Medical Association* (medication errors and ventilator-associated pneumonia)
- NICE (National Institute for Health and Care Excellence) guidelines, for example clinical guideline CG161 for falls, NG10 for violence, aggression, and bullying
- *Nursing Times* (needle stick injuries) and the *Journal of Mental Health* (violence, aggression, and bullying). Search for articles that discuss strengths and limitations of de-escalation and breakaway techniques
- Supporting managers and educators to develop healthcare support worker roles: see http://www.hcswtoolkit.nes.scot.nhs.uk

---

Table 5.11   Critique of methods used within education and training

	Strengths	Limitations
Journal clubs	Up-to-date research papers that focus on current practice can be explored	Requires commitment and motivation from individuals to read, summarize key points, and apply learning to practice
Simulations – for example, use of manikins, actors, computer programs	Interactive and engaging	Resource-intensive
Critical incident reviews/case study discussions	Current and relevant to teams, therefore stimulating and motivating	Need time for reflection and can therefore be time-consuming
Lectures	Can be delivered to large numbers	Take time to prepare, and lecturer may not engage the audience
Workshops	Generally hands on and interactive	Due to small numbers could be costly if need to be repeated

(Continues)

Table 5.11 (Continued)

E-learning/ distance learning	Undertaken at a convenient time and at individual's own pace	If participants do not engage in online discussions and debates, the learning process could be lonely and limited learning may occur
Private study	Undertaken at a convenient time and at individual's own pace	Requires motivation and commitment and good time management skills

Table 5.12 Accessing CPD opportunities via the internet

http://www.rcn.org.uk/development/learning/learningzone
- This will take you to the UK Royal College of Nursing website "Learning Zone"
- This is a useful website for healthcare assistants, assistant practitioners, and student and registered nurses who work in different settings
- Explore the varied opportunities that you have to engage in online continuing professional development (CPD)
- For example, you might be interested in engaging in learning activities in relation to patient safety or in supporting people's nutritional needs (relevant for pressure ulcers). You might also like to explore the guidance and legislation provided in relation to violence in the workplace and bullying and harassment in the workplace

http://www.cot.co.uk
- This will take you to the College of Occupational Therapy website
- Resources are provided that enable practitioners to engage in lifelong learning and CPD opportunities
- Resources include interactive e-learning, videos, and printable resources
- Members of the British Association of Occupational Therapists can access an Interactive Learning Opportunities Database (ILOD)

http://www.csp.prg.uk/professional-union/careers-development/cpd
- This will take you to the Chartered Society of Physiotherapy
- CPD opportunities are provided through a championing CPD project that facilitates peer support for CPD development of skills and knowledge in the workplace through Learning Champions

---

Activity 5.12

Previous activities asked you to consider methods that are used at the individual, team, and organizational levels to facilitate learning.

- Can you think of other methods?
- Table 5.11 provides one strength and one limitation. Reflect on these methods and consider further strengths and limitations.

Table 5.12 provides useful links to some profession-specific CPD opportunities that you might like to explore.

Key points summary

Education and training underpin the implementation of clinical governance strategies and is essential if the risks to patients' safety are to be kept to a minimum. Education can be both formal and informal and in a learning organization should take place at the individual, team, and organizational levels.

* It is both a personal and organizational responsibility that members of staff at all levels are engaged in CPD
* In order to be a learning organization, all members of staff will benefit from an annual appraisal or personal development review
* In order to take part in appropriate CPD activities, it is important for staff to understand their learning styles

Implications for practice

* A match of individual and organizational values will likely impact on the retention of staff
* Experienced staff need to be aware that new members of staff coming into their team may experience transition shock
* As autonomous practitioners, clinical staff have a personal responsibility to engage in CPD

End-of-chapter questions

1 What are the key differences between Schein's (2010) levels of culture?
2 Which is the most inclusive of Handy's (1999) four cultural types?
3 What is the disadvantage of this cultural type?

See the Appendix on page 254 for suggested answers to these questions.

References

Barr, J. and Dowding, L. (2012) *Leadership in Health Care*. London: Sage.
Brennan, G. and McSherry, R. (2006) Exploring the transition and professional socialisation from healthcare assistant to student nurse, *Nurse Education in Practice*, 7 (4): 206–214.

Brown, J., Stevens, J., and Kermonde, S. (2013) Measuring student nurse professional socialisation: The development and implementation of a new instrument, *Nurse Education Today*, 33 (6): 565–573.

Carnall, C. (2007) *Managing Change in Organisations*, 5th edition. Harlow: Prentice-Hall.

Daniel, J. (2012) Making sense of MOOCs: Musings in a maze of myth, paradox and possibility, *Journal of Interactive Media in Education*, 18. Available at: https://jime. open.ac.uk/articles/10.5334/2012-18/ (accessed: 7 March 2021).

Department of Health (1998) *A Ffirst Cclass Sservice: Quality in the new NHS*. London: Department of Health.

Department of Health (2012) *Liberating the NHS: Developing the healthcare workforce. From design to delivery*. Available at: https://www.gov.uk/government/uploads/ system/uploads/attachment_data/file/216421/dh_132087.pdf (accessed: 7 March 2021).

Department of Health (2013) *The Education Outcomes Framework*. Available at: https:// www.gov.uk/government/uploads/system/uploads/attachment_data/file/175546/Education_outcomes_framework.pdf (accessed: 7 March 2021).

Duchscher, J. (2009) Transition shock: The initial stage of role adaptation for newly graduated registered nurses, *Journal of Advanced Nursing*, 65 (5): 1103–1113.

Edwards, G. (2018) From policy to practice: The challenges facing Uganda in reducing maternal mortality, *International Journal of Health Governance*, 23 (3): 226–232.

Executive Agency for Health and Consumers (EAHC) (2013) *Study Concerning the Review and Mapping of Continuous Professional Development and Lifelong Learning for Health Professionals in the EU: Final report*, EAHC/2013/Health/07. Available at: https://ec.europa.eu/health/sites/health/files/workforce/docs/cpd_mapping_report_ en.pdf (accessed: 7 March 2021).

Fleming, N. (1987) A Guide to Learning styles VARK. Available at: https://vark-learn.com (accessed: 7 March 2021).

Gillett, K., Reed, L., and Bryan, L. (2017) Using action learning sets to support change in end-of-life care, *Leadership in Health Services*, 30 (2): 184–193.

Gopee, N. and Galloway, J. (2009) *Leadership and Management in Healthcare*. London: Sage.

Haith, M.P. (2012) How to use action learning sets to support nurses, *Nursing Times*, 108 (18/19): 12–14.

Handy, C. (1999) *Understanding Organisations*. London: Penguin.

Haywood, H., Pain, H., Ryan, S., and Adams, J. (2013) Continuing professional development: Issues raised by nurses and allied health professionals working in musculoskeletal settings, *Musculoskeletal Care*, 11 (3): 136–144.

Health and Care Professions Council (HCPC) (2018) *Continuing Professional Development*. Available at: https://www.hcpc-uk.org/cpd (accessed: 7 March 2012).

Hearle, D., Lawson, S., and Morris, R., (2016) *A Strategic Guide to Continuing Professional Development for Health and Care Professionals: The TRAMm Model*. Keswick: M&K Publishing.

Hofstede, G. (1968) *Culture Consequences*. Harmondsworth: Penguin.

Huczynski, A. and Buchanan, D. (2007) *Organizational Behaviour*. Harlow: Prentice-Hall.

Institute for Safe Medication Practices (ISMP) (2007) *The Five Rights: A destination without a map*. Available at: http://www.ismp.org/Newsletters/acutecare/ articles/20070125.asp (accessed: 7 March 2021).)

Jackson, C. and Thurgate, C. (eds.) (2011) *Workplace Learning in Health and Social Care: A student's guide*. Maidenhead: Open University Press.

James, A.H. and Stacey-Emile, G. (2019) Action learning: Staff development, implementing change, interdisciplinary working and leadership, *Journal of Nursing Management*, 26 (3): 36–41.

Johnson, G. (1988) Rethinking incrementalism, *Strategic Management Journal*, 9 (1): 75–91.

Kelemen, M. (2005) *Managing Quality*. London: Sage.

Mullins, L. (2010) *Management and Organisational Behaviour*. Harlow: Prentice-Hall.

NICE (2018) *NICE Guidance*. Available at: https://www.nice.org.uk/guidance (accessed: 7 March 2021).

Nurakynova, S. (2018) Medical education governance based on strategic planning: An example of Kazakhstan medical universities, *International Journal of Health Governance*, 23 (3): 216–225.

Pedlar, M. (2008) *Action Learning for Managers*. London: Routledge.

Reineck, C. (2002) Leadership's guiding light, part 2: Create a learning organisation, *Nursing Management*, 33 (10): 13–18.

Sale, D. (2005) *Understanding Clinical Governance and Quality Assurance: Making it happen*. Basingstoke: Palgrave Macmillan.

Schein, E.H. (2010) *Organizational Culture and Leadership*, 4th edition. San Francisco, CA: Jossey-Bass.

Swage, T. (2004) *Clinical Governance in Healthcare Practice*. London: Butterworth Heinemann.

Vásquez-Sánchez, M.A., Jiménez-Arcos, M., Aguilar-Trujillo, P., Guardiola-Cardenas, M., Damián-Jiménez, F., and Casals, C. (2020) Characteristics of recovery from near misses in primary health care nursing: A prospective descriptive study, *Journal of Nursing Management*, 28: 2007–2016.

Wright, J. and Hill, P. (2003) *Clinical Governance*. London: Churchill Livingstone.

6 How clinical governance can be supported through evidence-based practice and values-based practice

Gail E. Lansdown

Chapter contents

- Learning objectives
- Introduction
- Evidence-based practice
- Values-based practice
- Accountability
- The link between evidence-based practice, quality assurance, and clinical governance
- How to use the evidence: defining the problem using PICOT
- Finding evidence: accessing information

- Research methods
- Critically appraising the evidence
- Issues and challenges
- Evidence-based practice and integrated care pathways
- Evidence-based practice and care bundles
- Key points summary
- Implications for practice
- End-of-chapter questions
- References

Learning objectives

By the end of this chapter, the reader will have a better understanding of:

- Definitions of evidence-based practice (EBP) and values-based practice (VBP)

- The link between EBP/VBP, quality assurance, and clinical governance
- Using evidence – defining a problem with PICOT
- Accessing evidence and types of evidence – an overview of the research process
- Critically appraising the evidence
- The legal implications of EBP
- EBP and integrated care pathways
- EBP and care bundles

Introduction

The previous chapter focused on education and training. This chapter will focus on the importance of EBP and VBP and how they apply to clinical governance.

Evidence-based practice

Evidence-based practice (EBP) is a term that has gained much popularity in recent years. EBP is a movement towards an increased assimilation of newly generated research evidence into direct patient care delivery and has influenced the healthcare sector for more than two decades. However, it is a complex issue and has been defined and redefined many times.

Put simply, EBP is practice that is supported by a clear and up-to-date rationale, taking into account the patient's preferences and based on professional judgement. The term was coined by Sackett and his colleagues, who defined EBP as "the conscientious, explicit and judicious use of current best evidence in making decisions about the care of individual patients" (1996: 71). They asserted that good doctors – we now replace "good doctors" with good healthcare professionals – should use both their clinical expertise and skills and the best available evidence to provide the best care for their patients. They further stated that neither on their own – that is, evidence or care – is sufficient and that the best available evidence needs to be taken in context, in that it may be inappropriate for an individual patient. Equally, practice becomes outdated if there is no reference to current best evidence. Further than this, though, is the need to remember that EBP is not only an amalgamation of scientific evidence and clinical expertise, but also a reflection of patients' needs and choices.

Two of the criticisms of EBP, however, are that it "ties the hands of practitioners and robs patients of their personal choices in reaching a decision about optimal care" (DaCruz, 2002: 674). Haynes, Devereaux, and Guyatt (2002) dispute this, agreeing that there are barriers to EBP, but stating that these are not two of them. They state that clinical decisions must be based on the preference of patients. They posit that clinical decisions must include:

1 An understanding of the patient's clinical and physical condition in order to verify what is wrong and what treatments are available
2 Research evidence that highlights the efficacy, effectiveness, and efficiency of the possible treatments
3 Consideration of the patient's preferences
4 The recommendation of a treatment, which the patient accepts

So, as an example, the evidence-based prescription of anticoagulants to a patient with a risk from stroke will not be dictated merely by considering the positive effect of anticoagulation. The decision must also consider the adverse side effects and will vary from patient to patient according to their clinical and physical condition, in line with point 1 above. Additionally, any recommended treatment must be agreed with the patient, as stated in point 4 above.

Dawes *et al.* (2005: 2) offer a softer and more holistic definition of EBP:

> *Evidence based practice requires that decisions about healthcare are based on the best available current valid and relevant evidence. These decisions should be made by those receiving care, informed by the tacit and explicit knowledge of those providing care, within the context of available resources.*

Definitions of evidence-based nursing vary in the literature. Melnyk *et al.* (2008: 11) define EBP as

> *... a problem-solving approach to clinical practice that integrates a systematic search for, and critical appraisal of, the most relevant evidence to answer a burning clinical question, one's own clinical expertise, patient preferences and values.*

They state that evidence-based nursing practice involves the following steps:

- Asking a clinical question
- Searching for the best evidence
- Critically appraising the evidence
- Integrating the evidence with one's clinical expertise and patient preferences and values
- Evaluating the outcomes of practice decisions or changes based on evidence

Scott and McSherry's (2009: 1089) review of the literature led them to suggest the following definition:

> *An ongoing process by which evidence, nursing theory and the practitioner's clinical expertise are critically evaluated and considered, in conjunction with patient involvement, to provide delivery of optimum nursing care for the individual.*

Although the definition of EBP has evolved somewhat over time, there is agreement that the integration of best research evidence, individual clinical expertise, and patient choice is key.

Values-based practice

Ethical values are probably the most widely acknowledged values in health and social care. Values, however, are broader than ethics and include needs, wishes, preferences, and anxieties, to name but a few. Values are person-specific and culture-based. No discussion on EBP would be complete without a consideration of values-based practice (VBP), which has been defined by Woodbridge and Fulford (2003: 32) as:

> ... *putting the values of individual service users and carers at the centre of everything we do. It also means understanding and using our own values and beliefs in a positive way and respecting the values of the other people we work with.*

Fulford (2011) discusses the new partnership between EBP and VBP, illuminating the synergy between EBP and VBP in delivering care by incorporating a patient's values. Taking a step further than EBP, Fulford (2011) states that by incorporating a patient's unique values, such as preferences, anxieties, needs, and wishes into a decision based on clinical evidence leads to patient-centred medicine. However, Fernandez and Wieten (2015) add that the clinician's values must also be taken into account. It is equally important to remember that values, both those of the patient and the clinician, may change over time, particularly in patients with psychiatric disorders. Also of note is the fact that the values of patients and clinicians may potentially be in conflict (Mohanna, 2017).

VBP was initially predominantly embodied within the field of mental health at the Centre for Clinical and Academic Workforce Innovation (CCAWI, 2005) at the University of Lincoln. Subsequently, the CCAWI evolved into Research in Mental Health, Health and Social Care, or MH2aSC. Broadening the interests of CCAWI, MH2aSC contributes to government policy strategies as well as driving innovations in health and social care settings. Its key research themes include mental health, the integration of health and social care, VBP, workforce development, and service improvement.

Evolving policy and legislation to improve patient-centred care in mental health and the increasing imperative to include values, rights, and personal outcomes in care resulted in 10 Essential Shared Capabilities (ESC). A Department of Health-funded initiative to examine the application of VBP into partnerships with service users, carers, and others working in mental health (CCAWI, 2005), the 10 ESCs are:

1 Working in partnership
2 Respecting diversity

3 Practising ethically

4 Challenging inequality

5 Promoting recovery, wellbeing, and self-management

6 Identifying people's needs and strengths

7 Providing person-centred care

8 Making a difference

9 Promoting safety and risk enablement

10 Personal development and learning

Further detail regarding the 10 ESCs is given in the Department of Health (2004) framework for the mental health workforce. Appendix A of this document shows the link between ESCs, the Capable Practitioner Framework (CPF), the National Occupational Standards (NOS), and the Knowledge and Skills Framework (KSF). It is important to remember that the four frameworks were developed separately; they do not cover the same issues and the ESC, the CPF, and the NOS have been developed for mental health services, whilst the KSF has an NHS focus. Figure 6.1 illustrates how values, rights, and personal outcomes are incorporated in the improvement of patient-centred care.

The links below provide access to the frameworks:

Figure 6.1 Improving patient-centred care

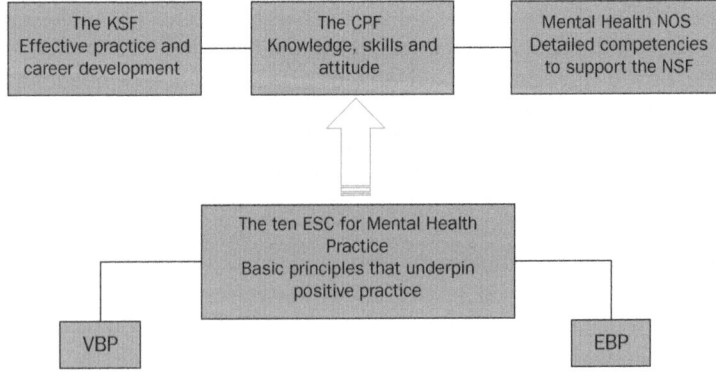

Adapted from: Woodbridge and Fulford (2003).

– *Knowledge and Skills Framework*
  https://www.evidence.nhs.uk/search?q=knowledge+skills+framework
  (accessed: 7 March 2021)

– *Capable Practitioner Framework*
  https://www.hee.nhs.uk/sites/default/files/documents/ACP%20Primary%20
  Care%20Nurse%20Fwk%202020.pdf (accessed: 7 March 2021)

– *National Occupational Standards*
  https://www.gov.uk/government/publications/national-occupational-standards
  (accessed: 7 March 2021)

Fulford (2011) adds to Figure 6.1 in stating that all clinical decisions stand on two feet: left foot = values, and right foot = evidence.

The National Institute for Mental Health England (NIMHE, 2004) lists the following principles of VBP:

- Recognition of the role of values alongside evidence in all areas of mental health delivery and practice
- Raising awareness that values are context-based, and the impact they have on practice in mental health
- Respect of the diversity of values, working to ensure that the principle of service-user centrality is the unifying focus for practice. By so doing, the values of each service user/client and their communities must be the key determinant of all actions taken by professionals

Respect for diversity is seen as:

- User-centred – the values of individual users are central
- Recovery-oriented – cultural and racial difference impact on the routes to recovery
- Multidisciplinary – respect is reciprocal at an individual level, at a disciplinary level (nursing, medicine, social work), and at an organizational level (health, social care, community groups, etc.)
- Dynamic – respect is responsive to change
- Balanced – positive and negative values are recognized
- Relational – positive working relationships supported by good communication at the heart of practice

Fulford, Carroll, and Peile (2011) suggest a 10-part process of value-based practice:

Four learnable clinical skills:
1 Awareness of values and how these may differ
2 Reasoning skills
3 Knowledge of values
4 Communication skills

An enabling clinical environment:
5 One is person-centred
6 The other multidisciplinary

Four specific links with EBP:
7 The two-feet principle
8 The squeaky wheel principle
9 The science-driven principle
10 Partnership between stakeholders

To explain further, the two-feet principle states that all decisions need to rest on values as well as evidence. The squeaky wheel principle suggests that we tend to notice values when they cause conflicts. The science-driven principle works on the fact that advances in treatment drive the need for both evidence-based practice and values-based practice because new choices are likely to affect values.

Wareing (2017) describes the Me, My, More, Must approach that can enable healthcare professionals to consider who they are and what impact their values might have on a particular situation (Table 6.1). He states that a values-based approach to healthcare materialized after several high-profile moral catastrophes, such as the poor standards of care at the Mid Staffordshire NHS Foundation Trust and the abuse of residents at the Winterbourne View unit. These and other such high-profile issues have supported reflection on values such as the 6Cs (compassion, caring, communication, competence, courage, and commitment) and have led to values-based reflection (Wareing, 2017).

Activity 6.1

- What key elements do all of the definitions of EBP have in common?
- Does this fit with your understanding of EBP?

Activity 6.2

Where do you think the balance should lie between the health or social care provider making a decision and that decision being made by those in receipt of care? Consider the legal, ethical, and professional responsibilities of the healthcare professional, for example paternalism vs. advocacy and patient autonomy, deontology vs. utilitarianism.

Activity 6.3

- Have you made a clinical decision recently?
- Regardless of whether you work in a mental health facility or not, was your decision based on the 10 ESCs and the NIMHE's three guiding principles?
- If not, how might you incorporate these into future clinical decision-making?
- Using the questions identified in Table. 6.1 from Wareing's (2017) Me, My, More, Must model, consider a clinical issue in which you were involved.

Table 6.1 The Me, My, More, Must model of values-based reflection

Stage	Writing prompt
Me	What values are important to me as a person? What values are important to me as a healthcare worker? What do I need in order to feel confident at work? What decreases my confidence at work? What enables me to be able to practise effectively in a clinical or therapeutic area? What prevents me from practising effectively in a clinical or therapeutic area?
My	What are my thoughts and feelings regarding this learning experience, situation, or incident? What concerns do I have regarding myself? What concerns do I have about other people involved in this experience? Who can help me make sense of this experience or situation? What impact have my values had on the people involved in this experience? What impact has my level of confidence had on how I have practised during this experience? In general, what have I learnt from this experience, situation, or incident?
More	What questions have been generated from this experience, situation, or incident? What ideas have been generated from this experience, situation, or incident? What has surprised or puzzled me about this experience, situation, or incident? What do I need to find out more about, as a result of this experience, situation, or incident?
Must	What must I do now to identify my learning needs? What must I do to identify my learning goals? Who must I speak to, to assist me in creating a learning or development plan? What must I include in the plan? What values must I explore in order to become the healthcare worker I wish to become?

Adapted from: Wareing (2017: 271).

Case study

You have planned to go on a remote trekking holiday in a country where malaria is prevalent. You attend a travel clinic to enquire about malaria prophylaxis. Unfortunately, the practitioner that you see is not up to date and recommends malaria prophylaxis that is now rarely used and is largely considered to be ineffective against modern strains of malaria.

Other more effective drugs with fewer adverse side effects are now prescribed for malaria prophylaxis. However, the practitioner has been administering this older drug for years and is unaware of the newer, more effective drugs. You take the older drug recommended by the practitioner.

The practitioner in the case study is not engaging in EBP because they are not using the best up-to-date evidence to inform their practice. As a result, the practitioner is putting your health at risk.

Accountability

As a healthcare professional you are accountable. This means that you have a professional responsibility to justify and give a clear account of, and rationale for, your practice. Failure to do this may result in professional misconduct. We are accountable not only to our professional body but are also accountable under the law.

Activity 6.4

As an accountable healthcare professional, what elements of your professional code of conduct support the use of EBP?

Could the practitioner in the case study above justify and give a clear account and rationale for their practice? Clearly, when you are called to account for your practice, you will only be able to justify it if you have administered care that is based on the best available evidence. You will not be able to account for care that is based on old or weak evidence.

If there were a standard or a policy document in the practitioner's place of work that recommended the newer malaria prophylaxis, then they would find it difficult to justify administering the old medication. Even if there was no such documentation or standard, the practitioner would still find it difficult to justify why an outdated medication was administered when a more effective one was available.

In summary, shared decision-making, or evidence-informed decision-making (EIDM), should be informed by the best available evidence, the patient's values, and, as far as possible, devoid of the clinician's bias or preferences. The following three points are essential in shared decision-making:

1 The clinician and patient agree that a decision is required
2 Both the clinician and the patient acknowledge and discuss the risks and benefits of all available treatment options
3 There needs to be an acknowledgement and discussion of the possible difference between the clinician's guidance and the patient's values and preferences.

Three barriers to involving patients in decision-making must also be recognized (Légaré et al., 2008):

1 Time constraints
2 A possible perception from clinicians that patient characteristics, such as educational level or socio-economic status, might preclude a meaningful discussion

3 The possibility that process or outcome targets that impact on a clinician's items for service payments, for example administration of the flu vaccine, might disincentivize clinicians from engaging with patients in joint decision-making

The link between evidence-based practice, quality assurance, and clinical governance

Quality is both a vision and an attribute in healthcare. We gave a number of definitions of quality in Chapter 1, but it is also important to remember that quality assurance in healthcare is also high on the global agenda.

The World Organization of Family Doctors for Asia (WONCA, 2005) define quality assurance as a process of planned activities based on performance review and enhancement with the aim of continually improving standards of patient care.

Quality assurance is a means of ensuring that practitioners are engaging in best practice, that their clinical decisions are based on current evidence, and that patients are receiving the best available care. It involves looking at the delivery of healthcare in your own practice through activities such as clinical audit, review of preventative care activities, surveys of patient satisfaction, and reviews of the practice of the organization. It is a way of identifying areas for further education or for making useful changes in practice.

In recent years, amidst other attempts, clinical governance has emerged to become an effective approach to pursuing quality of care. The UK National Health Service defined clinical governance as "a framework through which organisations are accountable for continuously improving the quality of their services and safeguarding high standards of care by creating an environment in which excellence in clinical care will flourish" (Department of Health, 1998: 33).

As discussed in Chapter 1, the key components of clinical governance are a comprehensive quality improvement programme, arrangements for continuing professional development, policies for managing risk and tackling poor performance, and clear lines of accountability for the quality of care.

Activity 6.5

Consider the case study above. How could clinical governance activities ensure that the practitioner administered the correct malaria prophylaxis?

Barría (2014) states that nursing research contributes to EBP by informing quality care, patient safety, and cost-effectiveness. Furthermore, EBP is a core competency requirement for nursing practice internationally (Fleiszer *et al.*, 2016). It has been shown that two of the barriers to EBP are lack of time and an unsupportive organizational culture. Bianchi *et al.* (2018) make the case that nurse managers and ward culture are barriers to EBP. In an analysis of 28 articles from a search of PubMed, CINAHL, and the Cochrane Library (2006–2016), they posit that nurse managers have an influential role in the implementation of EBP, and it is important that they foster a supportive culture and address the barriers to using evidence to support clinical decisions. In a Chinese study, Fu *et al.* (2020) highlight the barriers listed in Table 6.2.

Table 6.2 Barriers to EBP in China

Themes	Sub-themes
Evidence	Lack of evidence sources
	A gap between evidence and clinical context
Nurses	Lack of knowledge and skills in gathering evidence
	Increased workloads and poor compliance
Patients	Perceptions, attitudes, and knowledge
	Low compliance
Setting	Cultural barriers
	Mismatch with hospital needs, poor ward atmosphere
Support	Lack of leadership
	Lack of resources (finance, equipment)
	Lack of support from other healthcare professionals

Adapted from: Fu *et al.* (2020: 1040).

An article published by Melnyk *et al.* (2018) in the United States is much more concerning. In the first US study of nurses' EBP competencies, they demonstrate major deficits that threaten healthcare quality, safety, and patient outcomes. Their study was fuelled by the fact that, although the first set of competencies for nurses was published in 2014, no research has been undertaken to assess compliance. They found that of 2,344 nurses from 19 hospitals or healthcare facilities who were surveyed, not one of them had met any of the 24 competencies. They recommend that it is the responsibility of academic institutions to ensure that all graduates have EBP skills before graduation and healthcare organizations should require it as standard for all clinicians.

Litigation and negligence

Another reason why it is important that healthcare professionals can justify the care that they give is that this may protect themselves or the healthcare organization from litigation. As discussed previously, there is a developing culture of litigation and claims against healthcare organizations. Patients or clients who are unhappy about the care they receive can make a claim of negligence if they have suffered harm as a result of that care.

Activity 6.6

Consider the case study again. Imagine that the worst does occur and you contract malaria during your remote trek. You become very ill and are unable to work during your illness and recovery period. What laws are in place to protect you? How would the legal system support you in getting compensation?

How to use the evidence: defining the problem using PICOT

You will need to ask an answerable question if you are looking for evidence to inform your practice (to improve it, or to confirm that it is the best that it can be). Without a well-focused question, it can be very difficult and time-consuming to find relevant literature.

The PICOT tool (Polit and Beck, 2013) is useful to ensure that your question is answerable:

P   Patient or population
I   Intervention or indicator
C   Comparison or control
O   Outcome
T   Time

As an example, how can PICOT be used to help reduce falls in the hospitalized confused elderly (Table 6.3)? The question you ask could be: "For the older confused patient on bed rest, is fitting bed safety rails preferable to not fitting them in the interests of reducing injury?"

This question focuses on an intervention but sometimes we will be more interested in the meanings or perceptions of a particular group or community. For example, if we wanted to explore the attitude of carers to using safety rails for older people, then the PICOT would be as in Table 6.4. And the question becomes: "For the older confused patient on bed rest, what are the attitudes of carers for the fitting of bed rails?"

Using PICOT requires practice, but it will help you devise a clearly focused research question and will make your quest for relevant research much easier. Having established your question, you need to search systematically for current literature to answer it.

Activity 6.7

Use PICOT to formulate a question related to your practice.

Table 6.3 Using PICOT: 1

Framework item	Think about	Example
Patient, Problem, or Population	What are the patient's demographics, such as age, gender, ethnicity, socio-economic status? Or what is the problem type?	Older, confused patients on bed rest
Intervention	What type of intervention (action or treatment) is being considered?	Fitting bed rails
Comparison or Control	Is a comparison treatment to be considered?	Not fitting bed rails
Outcome or Objective	What would be the desired outcome? How can that outcome be measured?	A reduction in injuries
Time	Timeframe – not all questions will be time bound	

Table 6.4 Using PICOT: 2

Framework item	Think about	Example
Patient, Problem, or Population	What are the patient's demographics, such as age, gender, ethnicity, socio-economic status? Or what is the problem type?	Older, confused patients on bed rest
Intervention	What type of intervention (action or treatment) is being considered?	Fitting bed rails
Comparison or Control or Context	Is a comparison treatment to be considered?	Safety
Outcome or Objective	What would be the desired outcome? How can that outcome be measured?	The attitude of carers
Time	Timeframe – not all questions will be time bound	

Finding evidence: accessing information

The internet affords us access to a raft of information, but we need to learn how to access relevant academic sources. Ideally, before you access the databases available to you, it is wise to plan your search on paper.

Thinking about the older confused patient in the example above, you might wish to carry out a search on the effectiveness of drug therapy in the management of Alzheimer's disease.

***

Activity 6.8

What would be the PICOT for this topic?

***

The question you might ask is: "How effective is drug therapy in the management of Alzheimer's disease?"

This question has three key words/phrases:

1 Alzheimer's disease
2 Drug therapy
3 Management

Having determined your key words, think of synonyms (words that are the same as, or similar to, your key terms). Using a dictionary or thesaurus will help you do this. Using the Boolean method of searching for literature requires the use of key words, plus the words AND, OR, and NOT in combination and with a variety of other techniques, for example truncation.

Using the word OR prompts you to find key words that are similar to your first key word, for example Alzheimer's OR dementia. When AND is used, a search is narrowed, for example combining the key words Alzheimer's disease AND drug therapy will give fewer hits than merely using the phrase Alzheimer's disease. Truncation * helps expand a search. Depending on the search engine or database, the symbol may be *, ?, or #. Table 6.5 illustrates a Boolean search you might use to explore the literature in a systematic way to answer your question.

There are many databases available, for example:

- British Nursing Index (BNI): The Royal College of Nursing provides information on how to search the BNI at: http://www.rcn.org.uk/elibrary
- PubMed has extensive guidelines on how to search the database on its site: http://www.nlm.nih.gov/bsd/disted/pubmed.html
- The Cumulative Index to Nursing and Allied Health Literature (CINAHL) is useful for nurses and allied health professionals: http://www.cinahl.com
- The Cochrane Library provides independent high-quality evidence of healthcare decision-making. Cochrane Reviews provide systematic reviews of primary research and are internationally recognized as the highest standard in evidence-based healthcare and can be found at: http://www.cochrane.org

Much recent evidence is now available online through various websites, for example:

- NICE Guidelines
- HQIP (Health Care Quality Improvement Partnership)

- NHS England
- The World Health Organization
- The Centers for Disease Control and Prevention

Table 6.5 Example of a Boolean search

Alzheimer* disease	Drug Therap*	Manag*
Neurological Disorder*	Drug*	Treat*
Dementia	Medicat*	
Elderly Mental Health	Psychiatric Disorders – Drug Therap*	

There are also many websites that present recent evidence in the form of protocols and guidelines. Local health authorities also produce evidence-based protocols. Healthcare professionals need to be able to critically appraise these websites, guidelines, and protocols in order to ascertain their quality and usefulness to practice. The Appraisal of Guidelines for REsearch & Evaluation (AGREE) Instrument is a tool that assesses the methodological rigour and transparency in which a guideline is developed to address the issue of variability in guideline quality. Further information can be found at:

https://www.agreetrust.org/wp-content/uploads/2013/10/AGREE-II-Users-Manual-and-23-item-Instrument_2009_UPDATE_2013.pdf (accessed: 7 March 2021)

Recording your searching strategy

Once you have undertaken a systematic electronic literature search, you should have a reasonable selection of articles that are relevant to your research question. As mentioned above, it may be helpful to keep a record of your searching strategy and the key words you used so that you can demonstrate a systematic approach that is the most likely to yield relevant literature for your topic. If you are searching for articles of primary research but are failing to identify these, you should document this fact. It is more accurate to write "I did not find any literature on X" than to state categorically "there is no literature …".

What counts as evidence in EBP?

Take the following example of the many things we need to consider when searching for a pair of perfect shoes. I have a formal wedding to go to next month. And I need to buy a new pair of shoes. To do this, I will need a strategy to make sure the shoes I purchase are the right ones. I will need to think about a number of things:

- Are they within my budget? (Feasibility)
- Are they right for the purpose or occasion? (Appropriateness)

- Are they comfortable? (Effectiveness)
- Do I like them? (Meaningfulness)

Whether buying shoes or making a clinical decision, there are many things to consider. The same set of criteria – feasibility, appropriateness, effectiveness, and meaningfulness – may apply to a clinical scenario.

Let us consider the use of thrombo-embolic deterrent (TED) stockings in the post-operative prevention of deep-vein thrombosis (DVT). Research evidence suggests that TED stockings are cost-effective, convenient, and have minimal side effects, making them feasible, appropriate, and effective in the prevention of post-operative DVT. However, if the patient's experience (meaningfulness) of TED stockings is that they are tight and uncomfortable to wear and they thus refuse to wear them, the other three factors are compromised. EBP is therefore more complex than at first sight.

Types of evidence

So, what different types of evidence influence our choices? Does one type of evidence take precedence over another?

There are many different types of evidence available to underpin our clinical practice. Below is a brief discussion of research paradigms, ontology, epistemology, methodologies, and methods. Positivism/post-positivism and interpretivism/constructivism are two basic research paradigms.

It is important to understand how positivism has metamorphosed into post-positivism. The positivists believed in empiricism whereby observation and measurement were key to understanding the world so that it could be controlled and predicted. Using deductive reasoning, theories were advanced and tested. A radical rethink of research paradigms in the mid-twentieth century resulted in a new paradigm, that of post-positivism. Post-positivists assert that the way scientists think and work and the way we think as we go about our daily lives is not all that different. Scientific reasoning and common-sense reasoning are part of the same process. The difference is in degree rather than kind. Notwithstanding, researching in a post-positivist paradigm requires rigour.

As with all scientific endeavour, we need to become familiar with the language (see Table 6.6). And with the positivist/post-positivist and interpretivist/constructionist paradigms in mind, table 6.7 gives an overview of the philosopy

Table 6.6 The basic language of research

Paradigm	A philosophical way of thinking – a worldview
Ontology	What is reality?
Epistemology	How can we know reality?
Theoretical experience	What approaches can we use to acquire knowledge?
Methodology	What procedure can we use to acquire knowledge?
Method	What tools can we use to acquire knowledge?
Source	What data can we collect and from where?

Table 6.7 Paradigms, ontology, epistemology, theoretical perspectives, methodologies, and methods

Paradigm	Ontology: What is reality?	Epistemology: How can I know reality/knowledge?	Theoretical perspective: What approach can we use to get knowledge?	Methodology: What procedure can we use to acquire knowledge?	Method: What tools can we use to acquire knowledge?
Positivism	There is a single reality or truth (more realist)	Reality can be measured and hence the focus is on reliable tools to obtain that	Positivism; post-positivism	Experimental research; survey research	Usually quantitative, e.g. sampling; measurement and scaling; statistical analysis, questionnaire
Constructivist/ Interpretive	There is no single reality or truth Reality is created by individuals in groups (less realist)	Therefore, reality needs to be interpreted It is used to discover the underlying meaning of events and activities	Interpretivism (reality needs to be interpreted) + Phenomenology + Symbolic interaction + Hermeneutics + Critical enquiry + Feminism	Grounded theory; phenomenology; ethnography; heuristic enquiry; action research; discourse analysis; feminist standpoint research, etc.	Usually qualitative, e.g. qualitative interview/focus group; observation; case study; life history; narrative; theme identification, etc.

of research. Table 6.8 lists the assumptions associated with the paradigms in question.

Table 6.8 Assumptions of positivist and interpretivist paradigms

Philosophical assumption	Positivism/post-positivism	Interpretivism
Ontological assumption (the nature of reality)	Reality is objective and singular and separate from the researcher	Reality is subjective and multiple, as seen by the researcher
Epistemological assumption (what constitutes knowledge)	Researcher is independent of that being researched	Researcher interacts with that being researched
Axiological assumption (the role of values)	Research is value-free and unbiased	Researcher acknowledges that research is value-laden and biases are present
Rhetorical assumption (the language of research)	Researcher writes in a formal style and uses the passive voice, accepted quantitative terms, and set definitions	Researcher writes in an informal stye and uses the personal voice, accepted qualitative terms, and limited definitions
Methodological assumption (the process of research)	Process is deductive. Study of cause and effect with a static design (categories are isolated beforehand). Research is context-free. Generalizations lead to prediction, explanation, and understanding. Results are accurate and reliable through validity and reliability	Process is inductive. Study of mutual simultaneous shaping factors with an emerging design (categories are identified during the process). Research is context-bound. Patterns and/or theories are developed for understanding. Findings are accurate and reliable through verification

Reproduced from: Konstantin Kaminski (no date), University of Bath, UK.

Research methods

Quantitative research

Quantitative research is the systematic scientific investigation of quantitative properties of phenomena and their relationships (Polit and Beck, 2013). The objective of quantitative research is to develop and employ mathematical models, theories, and/or hypotheses pertaining to natural phenomena. The process of measurement is central to quantitative research because it provides the fundamental connection between empirical observation and the mathematical expression of quantitative relationships.

Quantitative methods (Polit and Beck, 2013) involve:

- The generation of models, theories, and hypotheses
- The development of instruments and methods for measurement
- Experimental control and manipulation of variables
- Collection of empirical data
- Modelling and analysis of data
- Evaluation of results

Table 6.9 lists some of the quantitative research designs available and their applications.

Table 6.9 Quantitative research designs and their applications

Type of design	Key focus and control of variables	Intervention applied?	Example	Common study designs
Descriptive	Observational; describe "what is"; variables not controlled	No	A description of teenagers' attitudes towards smoking	Comparative descriptive designs; cross-sectional designs; longitudinal studies
Correlational	Explores and observes relationships among variables; variables not controlled	No	A study of the relationship between IQ and clinical depression	Descriptive correlational designs; predictive designs; model-testing designs
Quasi-experimental	Tests for causality with suboptimal variable control; independent variable not manipulated	Yes	A study of the effect of an after-school physical activity programme on childhood obesity rates	Pre- and post-test designs; post-test only designs; interrupted times-series designs
Experimental	Tests causality with optimal variable control; independent variable is manipulated	Yes	A study of the effect of a new diet treatment plan on insulin levels in diabetes	Classic experimental designs; randomized designs; crossover designs; nested designs

---

Activity 6.9

Identify the key approaches of the following quantitative research methods. In addition, for each method, think of a possible study that could be carried out in your area of practice.

- Randomized control trial
- Quasi experiment
- Cohort study
- Survey/questionnaire

Qualitative research

The principle of all qualitative research is to explore the meaning of and develop in-depth understanding of the research topic as experienced by the participants of the research. Qualitative research seeks to understand human behaviour and the social processes in which we engage. Depth rather than breadth is the focus of qualitative research.

Table 6.10 lists some of the qualitative dimensions and their applications.

Table 6.10   Qualitative research designs and their applications

Dimensions	Focus	Data collection	Data analysis	Narrative form
Grounded theory	Develop a theory grounded in field data	Interviews with 20–30 to saturate categories and generate a theory	Open coding; axial coding; selecting coding; conditional matrix	Theory or theoretical model
Phenomenology	Understanding the essence of experiences about a phenomenon	Long interviews with up to 10 people	Statements; meanings; meaning themes; general description of experience	Description of the essence of the experience
Ethnography	Describing and interpreting a cultural or social group	Primarily observations and interviews with additional artefacts during extended time in the field (e.g. 6 months to a year)	Description; analysis; interpretation	Description of the cultural behaviour of a group or an individual

(Continues)

Table 6.10 (Continued)

Dimensions	Focus	Data collection	Data analysis	Narrative form
Case study	Developing an in-depth analysis of a single case or multiple cases	Multiple sources including documents, archival records, interviews, observations, physical artefacts	Description; themes; assertions	In-depth study of a case or cases
Narrative	Exploring the life of an individual	Exploring the life of an individual	Stories; epiphanies; historical content	Detailed picture of an individual's life

Adapted from: Clark and Cresswell (2014).

Activity 6.10

Identify the key approaches of the following qualitative research methods. In addition, for each method, think of a possible study that could be carried out in your area of practice.

- Grounded theory
- Ethnography
- Phenomenology
- Action research

Fineout-Overholt, Melnyck and Stillwell (2010) describe four sources of evidence: research, clinical experience, patient experience and information from the local context. Fineout-Overholt, Melnyck and Stillwell (2010) argue that although research evidence has been traditionally viewed as the gold standard, it is not certain, a contextual and static but is dynamic and eclectic and therefore on its own is not enough to inform clinical decisions effectively. Knowledge accrued from professional practice, patient/client experience and the local context is also valued in EBP. It is evident that sometimes the different sources of evidence make uncomfortable bedfellows; however, if person/patient centred care is to be a reality, an accord between different sources of evidence needs to be found.

Hierarchy of evidence

A hierarchy of evidence – or levels of evidence – is used to reflect the methodological rigour of studies (Table 6.11). A study assigned as level 1 evidence is considered the most rigorous and least susceptible to bias, while a study deemed to be level 8 evidence is considered the least rigorous and is more susceptible to bias.

Table 6.11 Hierarchy of evidence

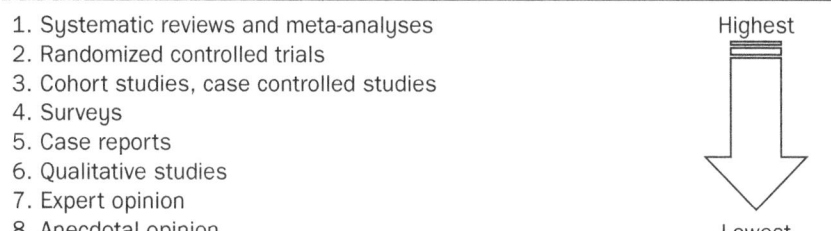

1. Systematic reviews and meta-analyses	Highest
2. Randomized controlled trials	
3. Cohort studies, case controlled studies	
4. Surveys	
5. Case reports	
6. Qualitative studies	
7. Expert opinion	
8. Anecdotal opinion	Lowest

There is general agreement that a hierarchy of evidence exists and that some forms of research evidence are stronger than others in addressing different types of questions. However, the hierarchy depends on the question you wish to have answered.

For example, if you wanted to find out whether the use of gloves was more effective than hand washing in the prevention of the spread of hospital-acquired infections, you would find stronger evidence from a randomized controlled trial that looked at a comparison between the two approaches than a study that asked the opinions of patients or clients as to which method they thought was more effective in preventing the spread of infection. The stronger evidence provided by the RCT in this instance indicates that the RCT should be placed higher up in a hierarchy than a study exploring patients' perception of hand hygiene when addressing this particular question.

In the hierarchy of evidence, the higher up a methodology is ranked, the more robust and close to objective truth it is assumed to be. One of the most well-known hierarchies of evidence that is concerned with ranking the strength of evidence relating to the effectiveness of a treatment or intervention is that developed by Sackett *et al.* (1996) as shown above.

However, it is also important to bear in mind that it is not always possible or desirable to undertake an RCT, even if this type of evidence is considered to be what is required. For example, for researchers looking at infant nutrition, it would not be acceptable or ethical to ask one group of mothers to abstain from breastfeeding their babies as a control for another group of mothers who were asked to breastfeed.

In many areas of health and social care, the traditional hierarchy is not appropriate for exploring complex questions. You are not only interested in finding out whether something is effective; there are many other questions you need to address.

Not all scholars agree with the approach of assigning a hierarchy of evidence. Some authors suggest that this approach is dangerous and may even subjugate nursing knowledge and practices.

Critically appraising the evidence

Once you have decided what you want to know and you have searched for evidence using an appropriate search strategy, you then need to weigh up how good the evidence is and what it means.

Critical appraisal has been described as the process of systematically examining research evidence to assess its validity, results, and relevance before using it to inform a decision (Hill and Spittlehouse, 2003). In order to do this, it is necessary to have a basic understanding of the different methodological approaches that may be taken within a research study, as this will help you to choose the correct critical appraisal tools.

The skills of critical appraisal are relatively easy to acquire and there are many tools to help you, but it is important to consider the most appropriate tools to use to appraise an individual piece of research critically. One study identified 121 published critical appraisal tools located on the internet and electronic databases (Katrak *et al.*, 2004). This raises the issue of which tool to use for a particular paper. Many critical appraisal tools have been developed for the review of specific types of research, and as such are design-specific, for example for the review of randomized controlled trials only. Other critical appraisal tools are generic and suitable for all types of research. At first glance, the reviewer might be tempted to use a critical appraisal tool that is generic to all types of research, especially if the literature searching strategy has identified many different approaches to research. However, the reviewer does need to assess the quality and appropriate application of the critical appraisal tool. Once you become engaged in the process, you will probably come to the conclusion that most research contains flaws but you will also be able to decide whether or not a piece of research has value in supporting your decision-making.

Tables 6.12 and 6.13 provide a step-by-step guide to critiquing quantitative and qualitative research, but as Katrak *et al.* (2004) noted, there are many from which to choose.

Table 6.12 Critiquing framework for quantitative research article

Elements	Questions
Writing style	Is the report well written – concise, grammatically correct, avoiding the use of jargon? Is it well laid out and organized?
Author	Do the researcher's qualifications/position indicate a degree of knowledge in this particular field?
Report title	Is the title clear, accurate, and unambiguous?
Abstract	Does the abstract offer a clear overview of the study including the research problem, sample, methodology, findings, and recommendations?

(Continues)

Table 6.12 (Continued)

Elements	Questions
Elements influencing the robustness of the research	
Purpose/research problem	Is the purpose of the study/research problem clearly identified?
Logical consistency	Does the research report follow the steps of the research process in a logical manner? Do these steps naturally flow and are the links clear?
Literature review	Is the review logically organized? Does it offer a balanced critical analysis of the literature? Is the majority of the literature of recent origin? Is it mainly from primary sources and of an empirical nature?
Theoretical framework	Has a conceptual or theoretical framework been identified? Is the framework adequately described? Is the framework appropriate?
Aims/objectives/ research question/ hypothesis	Have aims and objectives, a research question or hypothesis been identified? If so, are they clearly stated? Do they reflect the information presented in the literature review?
Sample	Has the target population been clearly identified? How was the sample selected? Was it a probability or non-probability sample? Is it of adequate size? Are the inclusion/exclusion criteria clearly identified?
Ethical considerations	Were the participants fully informed about the nature of the research? Was the autonomy/confidentiality of participants guaranteed? Were the participants protected from harm? Was ethical permission granted for the study?
Operational definitions	Are all the terms, theories, and concepts mentioned in the study clearly defined?
Methodology	Is the research design clearly identified? Has the data-gathering instrument been described Is the instrument appropriate? How was it developed? Was reliability and validity testing undertaken and the results discussed? Was a pilot study undertaken?
Data analysis/ results	What type of data and statistical analysis was undertaken? Was it appropriate? How many of the sample participated? Significance of the findings?
Discussion	Are the findings linked back to the literature review? If a hypothesis was identified, was it supported? Were the strengths and limitations of the study including generalizability discussed? Was a recommendation for further research made?
References	Were all the books, journals, and other media alluded to in the study accurately referenced?

Reproduced from: Coughlan *et al.* (2007).

Table 6.13 Critiquing framework for qualitative research article

Elements	Questions
Writing style	Is the report well written – concise, grammatically correct, avoiding the use of jargon? Is it well laid out and organized?
Author	Do the researcher's qualifications/position indicate a degree of knowledge in this particular field?
Report title	Is the title clear, accurate, and unambiguous?
Abstract	Does the abstract offer a clear overview of the study including the research problem, sample, methodology, findings and recommendations?
Elements influencing the robustness of the research	
Statement of the phenomenon of interest	Is the phenomenon to be studied clearly identified? Are the phenomenon of interest and the research question consistent?
Purpose/significance of the study	Is the purpose of the study/research question clearly identified?
Literature review	Has a literature review been undertaken? Does it meet the philosophical underpinnings of the study? Does the review of the literature fulfil its objectives?
Theoretical framework	Has a conceptual or theoretical framework been identified? Is the framework adequately described? Is the framework appropriate?
Method and philosophical underpinnings	Has the philosophical approach been identified? Why was this approach chosen? Have the philosophical underpinnings of the research been explained?
Sample	Is the sampling method and sample size identified? Is the sampling method appropriate? Were the participants suitable for informing research?
Ethical considerations	Were the participants fully informed about the nature of the research? Was the autonomy/confidentiality of participants guaranteed? Were the participants protected from harm? Was ethical permission granted for the study?
Data collection/data analysis	Are the data collection strategies described? Are the strategies used to analyse the date described? Did the researcher follow the steps of the data analysis method identified? Was data saturation achieved?
Rigour	Does the researcher discuss how rigour was assured? Were credibility, dependability, transferability, and goodness discussed?

(Continues)

Table 6.13 (Continued)

Elements	Questions
Findings/discussion	Are the findings presented appropriately? Has the report been placed in the context of what was already known of the phenomenon? Has the original purpose of the study been adequately addressed?
Conclusions/ implications and recommendations	Are the importance and implications of the findings identified? Are recommendations made to suggest how the research findings can be developed?
References	Were all the books, journals, and other media alluded to in the study accurately referenced?

Reproduced from: Coughlan *et al.* (2007).

Another useful link is to CASP (Critical Appraisal Skills Programme):

https://casp-uk.net/casp-tools-checklists/ (accessed: 7 March 2021)

where critiquing frameworks for the following are provided:

- Systematic reviews
- Randomized controlled trials
- Cohort studies
- Case control studies
- Economic evaluations
- Diagnostic studies
- Qualitative studies
- Clinical prediction rule

Issues and challenges

Since the 1990s, EBP has moved rapidly from a niche interest to a mainstream initiative, but does the reality match the theory and what are the issues that could prevent its full implementation? If we can understand these, then we may be able to find ways of overcoming them.

As discussed earlier in this chapter, there are many drivers for EBP, including the clinical governance and quality agenda as well as the need to follow the NMC Code of Professional Conduct and Code of Ethics for nurses. The Healthcare Professions Council (HCPC) lays out the Code of Conduct for paramedics; the Chartered Society of Physiotherapists (CSP) lays out the Code of Conduct for physiotherapists; the College of Occupational Therapists (COT) provides the Code of Ethics for occupational therapists; and the College of Operating Department Practitioners (HCPC) provides the Code for operating department practitioners. These drivers often require the healthcare professional to challenge traditional practice as well as outdated policies and guidelines.

Activity 6.11

You have had an outbreak of Norovirus in your clinical area and are aware that the most effective way of preventing further spread of infection is through hand washing. Your nursing colleagues wash their hands between patients; however, you notice that the doctors are not attending to this simple measure. How will you address this in the interests of effective patient care?

Legal implications of evidence-based practice

Pearson, Field, and Jordan (2007) argue that as we have declared that our past practice was not based on evidence and now the EBP movement has become unstoppable, the law is taking an increasing interest in seeing that the best care is provided for patients. Clinical negligence costs represent a major threat to the viability of the NHS, which paid £2.4bn (€2.8bn; $3.1bn) in clinical negligence claims in 2018–2019 according to NHS Resolution (2019) (formerly the NHS Litigation Authority). This sum is equivalent to about 2% of the NHS budget in England (Office of National Statistics, 2018). Errors during maternity care accounted for 50% of the total value of claims in 2018–2019, although only 10% of total claims (House of Commons Committee of Public Accounts, 2019). With approximately 600,00 births every year, the NHS pays approximately £12.7m per week for the cost of obstetric harm (Dyer, 2019). But this is not the full picture, and the amount set aside for claims is among the most substantial public sector financial liability. Yau *et al.* (2020) propose four principles to keep patients safe and reduce the number of claims:

1 Investing in staffing and infrastructure
2 A real commitment to learning
3 Learning from high performance
4 Enabling and supporting system-wide safety improvements, whereby quality improvement and methods such as plan-do-study-act cycles are no longer simply local but rather system-wide improvements

---

Activity 6.12

Do you believe that practice that is not deemed to be best practice ought to be regarded as negligent practice?

Feasibility, appropriateness, and meaningfulness

Feasibility, appropriateness, and meaningfulness are important and have been outlined by Pearson *et al.* (2007), reminding us that a further aspect of weighing up the value of a piece of research is to consider the patient or population we are most interested in.

Patient values, preferences, cultural and religious beliefs, as discussed previously in the section on values-based practice, will impact on the choice of an intervention we might offer patients in our role as healthcare practitioners.

Evidence and patient preference

As has been discussed earlier in this chapter, it is very important to consider the importance of patient preference in EBP. For example, a certain calcium alginate dressing may have stronger evidence for its use than another. However, an individual patient may prefer the alternative dressing because it results in less exudate and therefore means that the dressing is more manageable in everyday life. No matter how strong the evidence is, that patient is likely to take the dressing off when they get home and apply their own remedy. This will result in increased cost to whoever is paying for the wasted dressing and will also mean that you are spending time on carrying out needless dressings. Whatever the evidence suggests, consideration of the patient's preferences and the recommendation of a treatment that is acceptable to the patient are central to EBP and VBP.

In summary, Burns and Grove describe nursing research (to search again or to examine carefully) as a systematic and scientific inquiry that "… validates and refines existing knowledge and develops new knowledge that directly and indirectly influences nursing practice. Nursing research is the key to building an evidence based practice for nurses" (2011: 4).

The ultimate goal therefore is the "development of an empirical body of knowledge for a discipline or profession, such as nursing" (Burns and Grove, 2011: 4). In order for all healthcare professionals to promote positive outcomes for patients and their families, they need to be able to read and understand research reports to implement evidence-based practice. Often this evidence will be used to formulate protocols and guidelines.

The goal of EBP is to promote quality and cost-effective outcomes for patients, their families, and healthcare providers. As stated above, EBP is the integration of the best research evidence, clinical expertise, and patient needs and values through the application of VBP. The best research evidence is the empirical evidence that is generated from the synthesis of research findings to understand a problem in practice. Healthcare professionals require a solid research base in order to implement interventions to treat conditions and promote positive outcomes for both the patient and their family. In so doing, they will also ascertain that their patients receive quality care (Burns and Grove, 2011).

Evidence-based practice and integrated care pathways

Integrated care pathways were briefly mentioned in Table 1.2 (see page 15) when the attributes of clinical governance were first discussed. EBP is central to the formulation of care pathways and care bundles.

Terminology varies and integrated care pathways (ICP), anticipated recovery pathways (ARP), multidisciplinary pathways of care (MPC), collaborative care programmes (CCP) are terms that are used interchangeably. Swage (2004: 134) defines a care pathway as follows:

> An integrated care pathway determines locally agreed, multidisciplinary practice based on guidelines and evidence where available, for a specific patient/client group. It forms all or part of the clinical record, documents the care given and facilitates the evaluation of outcomes for continuous quality improvements.

Care pathways can provide patients with clear expectations of their care and are a means of measuring their progress; therefore, they can be seen to maximize the quality provided at each step of the patient's journey.

They also promote teamwork through an increased understanding of the differing roles of the multidisciplinary team. Additionally, they facilitate the use of guidelines (Evans-Lacko et al., 2010). For a specific patient group, a care pathway considers and maps all anticipated elements of care and all treatment provided by a multidisciplinary team of clinicians. Deviation from the pathway is noted in the patient's case notes as a variance, and variance analysis provides information on current practice. Furthermore, variance analysis encourages a multidisciplinary audit, as the team are able to analyse what care was actually given compared to the care that was laid down by the care pathway. The benefits of care pathways are numerous. However, teams also need to consider their limitations. Table 6.14 provides a critique of integrated care pathways.

A well-written pathway can lead to consistent care of the highest quality, thus supporting the notion of clinical governance. In order to be consistent there are a number of steps that need to be included when designing a pathway (Moullin, 2002; Swage, 2004; Sale, 2005):

- Identify patient group
- Set start/finish point (for example, admission and discharge; follow up to outpatients)
- Agree outcomes and personnel responsible
- Agree timescales
- Ensure that dates are recorded
- Track variances and analyse data

- Feedback and review
- Update pathway if necessary

Table 6.14   Critique of integrated care pathways

Benefits of pathways	Limitations of pathways
• Integrating evidence-based clinical guidelines into practice • Monitoring standards • Measuring quality • Some evidence that ICPs increase patient satisfaction • Involving all members of the multidisciplinary team • Reducing duplication • Improving consistency • Managing risk • Ensuring that treatment is evidence-based • Can be used as part of audit • Considered an audit-friendly tool • Can be used to identify where there are delays in the service • Standardized and therefore can reduce variations in service provided • Some evidence on the benefits of ICPs (RCTs) • Reduce hospital complications • Reduce hospital length of stay • Improve outcomes • Reduce costs • Avoid replication of care	• Lack of engagement of the organization, management, and clinical staff • It would appear that the greatest barrier is presented by clinical staff (Evans-Lacko *et al.*, 2010), who may be reluctant to change • Take time to design • Could be considered inflexible • Could be considered to prevent clinical decision-making • If electronic, computer problems • Difficult to design for an individual with multiple pathologies • Require leadership and good communication to implement successfully • Lack of evidence-based guidelines

Adapted from: Pickering and Thompson (2003), Swage (2004), Sale (2005), Allen *et al.* (2009), Rotter *et al.* (2008).

As stated above, there are limitations to integrated care plans (ICPs). One such example is the Liverpool Care Pathway for the Dying Patient (LCP). Whilst being endorsed by successive governments in England, the pathway was discontinued in 2014 following criticism and a national review.

It is also important to remember that integrated care pathways are not only workflow models but also records of care, which makes them both management and clinical tools, and this dichotomy can lead to tensions. Furthermore, tensions can also arise due to the fact that ICPs are about evidence-based practice plus quality improvement, the scientific knowledge of the former taking time to accumulate versus the urgency of implementation and feedback into practice (Seymour and Clark, 2018).

Resources

Bandolier provides further information on the use of integrated care pathways.
http://www.bandolier.org.uk/booth/glossary/ICP.html

The College of Occupational Therapy. If you type "pathways" into the search box on their website, you will find a number of pathways.
http://www.cot.co.uk

Lincolnshire Care Pathway Partnership. Here you will find an integrated pathway for MRSA.
http://mrsaactionuk.net/Lincs%20Care%20Pathway%20Project.pdf

Evidence-based practice and care bundles

It is essential for those working in critical care to ensure that their practices are evidence-based (Lawrence and Fulbrook, 2011), with the purpose of EBP being that existing evidence is applied to practice.

There are many forms of evidence and equally there are many ways in which evidence can be applied to practice; for example, the development of evidence-based protocols or care pathways, as discussed above. Building on this, Fulbrook and Mooney first described care bundles in the critical care nursing literature, describing a care bundle as follows: "the idea is that several practices, when used in combination, or as a cluster, all of the time, have a greater effect on the positive outcome of patients" (2003: 250).

Care bundles are a collection of interventions (usually three to five) that may be applied to the management of a particular condition. Based on evidence, the elements in a bundle are best practices brought together into a single quality measure (Aboelela, Stone, and Larson, 2007). We discussed ventilator-associated pneumonia (VAP) in Chapter 2, and Lawrence and Fulbrook (2011) suggest that a reduction in VAP is associated with VCB (ventilator care bundle) use and represents best practice for all eligible adult ventilated patients in intensive care.

Resources

High impact intervention – Care bundle to reduce ventilation-association pneumonia:
http://tinyurl.com/m2aw6qz (accessed: 7 March 2021)

Berenholtz, Dorman, and Provonost (2002) hypothesized the notion of bundling a number of interventions, with each intervention being based on strong evidence. They reviewed the literature between 1964 and 2000 and identified six outcome measures and six process measures that provided a measure of quality of intensive care. Four of the measures were grouped together by the Joint Commission on Accrediting of Healthcare Organizations (JCAHO) to form the VAP VCB:

1 Elevation of the head of the bed
2 Daily interruption of sedation to assess readiness to wean
3 Gastric ulcer prevention
4 Deep vein thrombosis prophylaxis (DVTP)

The four elements of Berenholtz and colleagues' (2002) VCBs were based on highest-level evidence, that is, systematic reviews of randomized control trials (RCTs) and single RCTs.

The VCB was tested in a 14-bed ICU for one year (Berenholtz *et al.*, 2004) and showed a decreased mortality if all four elements were applied. The Institute of Health Improvement conducted a multi-centre study in ICUs in the USA and Canada from 2002 to 2004, investigating the relationship between compliance with the VCB and its effect on clinical outcomes (O'Keefe-McCarthy, Santiago, and Lau, 2008). The study was significant because it demonstrated that VCB reduced ventilator days and ICU length of stay as well as dramatically reducing VAP rates.

Other research (DuBose *et al.*, 2008; Khorfan, 2008) has suggested adding oral care to the original four elements. Lawrence and Fulbrook (2011) were unable to prove the link between VCB and VAP incidence and length of ventilation and ICU length of stay, but a strong relationship is suggested.

Smith *et al.* (2020) have identified 21 studies on care bundles used in critically ill patients with COVID-19. Data, of course, are limited and based on observational clinical improvement. Research is urgently needed to develop care bundles that can be used collectively and consistently.

Resources

Pressure ulcer prevention and management care bundle:
https://sthelensccg.nhs.uk/media/3376/cheshire-merseyside-region-al-pressure-ulcer-core-policy-v10.pdf

FallSafe care bundles:
https://www.rcplondon.ac.uk/guidelines-policy/fallsafe-resources-original

---

Activity 6.13

- Have you used either an integrated care pathway or a care bundle?
- How helpful was it?

Key points summary

EBP and VBP are fundamental to improving clinical practice. A necessary part of EBP is to define a problem, preferably using PICOT, and access information (or evidence) in order to address the problem.

- Integrated care pathways, whilst not essential, enable multidisciplinary teams to work together to provide excellent patient care at each stage of the patient's journey. ICPs highlight variance that should be identified through audit. They also provide information to patients/service users on how their treatment will be managed
- Care bundles are a collection of interventions that can be applied to the management of a particular condition

Implications for practice

- All healthcare professionals must be accountable for their practice, and best practice includes appreciating the evidence
- Staff need to be aware of the limitations of integrated care pathways and care bundles

End-of-chapter questions

1 Why are EBP and VBP essential to clinical practice?
2 What is the difference between an integrated care pathway and a care bundle?
3 When examining your practice, what tool can help you ask an answerable question to ensure your practice is evidence-based?
4 What do the letters PICOT stand for?

See the Appendix on page 255 for suggested answers to these questions.

References

Aboelela, S.W., Stone, P.W., and Larson, L. (2007) Effectiveness of bundled behavioural interventions to control healthcare-associated infections: A systematic review of the literature, *Journal of Hospital Infection*, 66 (2): 101–108.

Allen, D., Gillen, E., and Rixon, L. (2009) Systematic review of the effectiveness of integrated care pathways: What works, for whom, in what circumstances?, *International Journal of Evidence-based Healthcare*, 7 (2): 61–74.

Barría, P. (2014) Implementing evidence-based practice: A challenge for the nursing practice, *Nursing Research and Education*, 32 (2): 191–193.

Berenholtz, S.M., Dorman, T., Ngo, K., and Provonost, P.J. (2002) Qualitative review of intensive care quality indicators, *Journal of Critical Care*, 17 (1): 1–12.

Berenholtz, S.M., Milanovich, S., Faircloth, A., Prow, D.I., Earsing, K., Lipsett, P. *et al.* (2004) Improving care for the ventilated patient, *Joint Commission Journal on Quality and Safety*, 30 (4): 195–204.

Bianchi, M., Bagnasco, A., Bressan, V., Barisone, M., Timmins, F., Rossi, S. *et al.* (2018) A review of the role of nurse leadership in promoting and sustaining evidence-based practice, *Journal of Nursing Management*, 26 (8): 918–932.

Burns, N. and Grove, S.K. (2011) *Understanding Nursing Research: Building an evidence based practice*, 5th edition. Maryland Heights, MO: W.B. Saunders.

Centre for Clinical and Academic Workforce Innovation (CCAWI) (2005) Available at: www.lincoln.ac.uk/xx_Archive/ccawi/ (accessed: 7 March 2021).

Clark, V.L.P. and Creswell, J.W. (2014) *Understanding Research: A consumer's guide.* London: Pearson Higher Education.

Coughlan, M., Cronin, P., and Ryan, F. (2007) Step-by-step guide to critiquing research. Part 1: quantitative research, *British Journal of Nursing*, 16 (11): 658–663.

Da Cruz, D. (2002) You have a choice dear patient, *British Medical Journal*, 324: 674.

Dawes, M., Summerskill, W., Glasziou, P., Cartabellotta, A., Martin, J., Hopayian, K. *et al.* (2005) Sicily statement on evidence-based practice, *BMC Medical Education*, 5: 1. Available at: https://doi.org/10.1186/1472-6920-5-1.

Department of Health (1998) *A First Class Service: Quality in the new NHS.* London: Department of Health.

Department of Health (2004) *The Ten Essential Shared Capabilities: A framework for the whole of the mental health workforce.* London: Department of Health.

DuBose, J.J., Inaba, K., Shiflett, A., Trankiem, C., Teixeira, P.G.R., Salim, A. *et al.* (2008) Measurable outcomes of quality improvement in the trauma intensive care unit: The impact of a daily quality rounding checklist, *Journal of Trauma, Injury, Infection and Critical Care*, 64 (1): 22–29.

Dyer, C. (2019) Government considers legal reforms to resolve high cost of clinical negligence claims, *British Medical Journal*, 364: l1362. Available at: https://doi.org/10.1136/bmj.l1362.

Evans-Lacko, S., Jarrett, M., McCrone, P., and Thornicroft, G. (2010) Facilitators and barriers to implementing clinical care pathways, *BMC Health Services Research*, 110: 82. Available at: https://doi.org/10.1186/1472-6963-10-182.

Fernandez, A.V. and Wieten, S. (2015) Values-based practice and phenomenological psychopathology: Implications of existential changes in depression, *Journal of Evaluation in Clinical Practice*, 21 (3): 508–513.

Fleiszer, A.R., Semenic, S., Ritchie, J.A., Richer, M.C., and Denis J.L. (2016) Nursing unit leaders' influence on the long-term sustainability of evidence-based practice improvements, *Journal of Nursing Management*, 24 (3): 309–318.

Fu, Y., Wang, C., Hu, Y., and Muir-Cochrane, E. (2020) The barriers to evidence-based nursing implementation in mainland China: A qualitative content analysis, *Nursing and Health Sciences*, 22 (4): 1038–1046.

Fulbrook, P. and Mooney, S. (2003) Care bundles in critical care: A practical approach to evidence-based practice, *Nursing in Critical Care*, 8 (6): 249–255.

Fulford, K.W.M. (2011) The value of evidence and evidence of values: Bringing together values-based and evidence-based practice in policy and service development in mental health, *Journal of Evaluation Clinical Practice*, 17 (5): 976–987.

Fulford, K.W.M., Carroll, H. and Peile, E. (2011) Values-based practice: Linking science with people, *Journal of Contemporary Psychotherapy*, 41 (3): 145–156.

Haynes, R.B., Devereaux, P.J., and Guyatt, G.H. (2002) Physicians' and patients' choices in evidence-based practice, *British Medical Journal*, 324: 1350. Available at: https://doi.org/10.1136/bmj.324.7350.1350.

Hill, A. and Spittlehouse, C. (2003) *Evidence Based Medicine: What is critical appraisal?* London: Hayward Medical Communications.

House of Commons Committee of Public Accounts (2019) *Managing the Costs of Clinical Negligence in Hospital Trusts, Fifth report of session 2017–19* (HC397). Available at: https://publications.parliament.uk/pa/cm201719/cmselect/cmpubacc/397/397.pdf (accessed: 7 March 2021).

Katrak, P., Bialocerkowski, A.E., Massy-Westropp, N., Kumar, V.S.S., and Grimmer, K.A. (2004) A systematic review of the content of critical appraisal tools, *BMC Medical Research Methodology*, 4: 22. Available at: https://doi.org/10.1186/1471-2288-4-22.

Khorfan, F. (2008) Daily goals checklist – a goal directed method to eliminate nosocomial infection in the intensive care unit, *Journal for Healthcare Quality*, 30 (6): 13–17.

Lawrence, P. and Fulbrook, P. (2011) The ventilator care bundle and its impact on ventilator-associated pneumonia: A review of the evidence, *Nursing in Critical Care*, 15 (5): 222–234.

Légaré, F., Ratté, S., Gravel, K., and Graham, I.D. (2008) Barriers and facilitators to implementing shared decision-making in clinical practice: Update of a systematic review of health professionals' perceptions, *Patient Education Counselling*, 73 (3): 526–535.

Melnyk, B.M., Fineout-Overholt, E., Feinstein, N.F., Sadler, L.S., and Green-Hernandez, C. (2008) Nurse practitioner educators' perceived knowledge, beliefs, and teaching strategies regarding evidence-based practice: Implications for accelerating the integration of evidence-based practice into graduate programs, *Journal of Professional Nursing*, 24 (1): 7–13.

Melnyk, B.M., Gallagher-Ford, L., Zellefrow, C., Tucker, S., Thomas, B., Sinnott, L.T. *et al.* (2018) The First U.S. study on nurses' evidence-based practice competencies indicates major deficits that threaten healthcare quality, safety, and patient outcomes, *World Views on Evidence-Based Nursing*, 15 (1): 16–25.

Mohanna, K. (2017) Values based practice: A framework for thinking with, *Education for Primary Care*, 28 (4): 192–196.

Moullin, M. (2002) *Delivering Excellence in Health and Social Care*. Maidenhead: Open University Press.

NHS Resolution (2019) *Annual Report and Accounts 2018/19*. Available at: https://assets.publishing.service.gov.uk/government/uploads/system/uploads/attachment_data/file/824345/NHS_Resolution_Annual_Report_and_accounts_print.pdf (accessed: 7 March 2021).

National Institute for Mental Health in England (NIMHE) (2004) *The Ten Essential Shared Capabilities: A framework for the whole of the mental health workforce*. Available at: https://webarchive.nationalarchives.gov.uk/20121102194627/http://www.dh.gov.uk/prod_consum_dh/groups/dh_digitalassets/@dh/@en/documents/digitalasset/dh_4087170.pdf (accessed: 6 July 2021).

Office for National Statistics (ONS) (2018) *Wider Measures of Public Sector Debt*. Available at: https://www.ons.gov.uk/economy/governmentpublicsectorandtaxes/publicsectorfinance/articles/widermeasuresofpublicsectornetdebt/december2018 (accessed: 7 March 2012).

O'Keefe-McCarthy, S., Santiago, C., and Lau, G. (2008) Ventilator-associated pneumonia bundled strategies: An evidence-based practice, *Worldviews on Evidence-Based Nursing*, 5 (4): 193–204.

Pearson, A., Field, J., and Jordan, Z. (2007) *Evidence-Based Clinical Practice in Nursing and Health Care: Assimilating research, experience and expertise*. Oxford: Blackwell.

Pickering, S. and Thompson, J. (2003) *Clinical Governance and Best Value*. London: Churchill Livingstone.

Polit, D.F. and Beck, C.T. (2013) *Essentials of Nursing Research: Appraising evidence for nursing practice*. Philadelphia, PA: Lippincott, Williams & Wilkins.

Rotter, T., Kugler, J., Koch, R., Gothe, H., Twork, S., Van Oostrum, J. *et al.* (2008) A systematic review and meta-analysis of the effects of clinical pathways on length of stay, hospital costs and patient outcomes, *BMC Health Services Research*, 8:. 265. Available at: https://doi.org/10.1186/1472-6963-8-265.

Sackett, D.L., Rosenberg, W.M., Muir Gray, J.A., and Richardson, W.S. (1996) Evidence based medicine: What it is and what it isn't, *British Medical Journal*, 312: 71. Available at: https://doi.org/10.1136/bmj.312.7023.71.

Sale, D. (2005) *Understanding Clinical Governance and Quality Assurance: Making it happen*. Basingstoke: Palgrave Macmillan.

Scott, K. and McSherry, R. (2009) Evidence-based nursing: Clarifying the concepts for nurses in practice, *Journal of Clinical Nursing*, 18 (8): 1085–1095.

Seymour, J. and Clark, D. (2018) The Liverpool Care Pathway for the Dying Patient: A critical analysis of its rise, demise and legacy in England, *Wellcome Open Research*, 3: 15. Available at: https://doi.org/10.12688/wellcomeopenres.13940.2.

Smith, V., Devane, D., Nichol, A., and Roche, D. (2020) Care bundles for improving outcomes in patients with COVID-19 or related conditions in intensive care – a rapid scoping review, *Cochrane Database of Systematic Reviews*, 12: CD013819. Available at: https://www.cochranelibrary.com/cdsr/doi/10.1002/14651858.CD013819/full (accessed: 25 June 2021).

Swage, T. (2004) *Clinical Governance in Health Care Practice*. Oxford: Butterworth Heinemann.

Wareing, M. (2017) Me, my, more, must: A values-based model of reflection, *Reflective Practice*, 18 (2): 268–279.

Woodbridge, K. and Fulford, K.W.M. (2003) Good practice? Values based practice in mental health, *Mental Health Practice*, 7 (2): 30–33.

World Organization of Family Doctors for Asia (WONCA) (2005) *Quality Assurance*. Available at: http://www.pdqa.gov.hk/english/qa/qa.php (accessed: 7 March 2021).

Yau, C.W.H., Leigh, B., Liberati, E., Punch, D., Dixon-Woods, M., and Draycott, T. (2020) Clinical negligence costs: Taking action to safeguard NHS sustainability, *British Medical Journal*, 368: m552. Available at: https://doi.org/10.1136/bmj.m552.

7 Implementing clinical governance through risk and complaints management

Gail E. Lansdown

Chapter contents

Learning objectives

By the end of this chapter, the reader will have a better understanding of:

- Quality control (QC), quality assurance (QA), total quality management (TQM), and continuous quality improvement (CQI)
- Clinical risk
- Risk management cycle: risk identification, analysis, control, and evaluation
- Complaints management, local resolution, independent review

- Learning from complaints
- Empowering patients/service users and staff to enable them to shape governance strategies collaboratively (shared governance)

Introduction

Chapter 5 introduced the concept of implementing clinical governance strategies through education and training. This chapter will focus on quality control and the use of risk management and complaints management to implement clinical governance.

Quality control, quality assurance, total quality management, and continuous quality improvement

Quality control is key in clinical governance, and it is widely believed that there are four approaches to quality:

1 Quality control (QC)
2 Total quality management (TQM)
3 Continuous quality improvement (CQI)
4 Quality assurance (QA)

We now look at each approach in turn.

Quality control

Let's begin by thinking back to Som's definition (2004: 89) of quality control:

> A governance system for healthcare organisations that promotes an integrated approach towards management of inputs, structures and processes to improve the outcome of the healthcare service delivery where health staff work in an environment of greater accountability for clinical quality.

The fundamentals of quality control have been in evidence, either directly or indirectly, for centuries. The Greeks and Egyptians set standards in their construction, arts, and crafts. In the Middle Ages and up to the nineteenth century, goods were manufactured in the main by individuals or small groups and so the notion of operator quality control was coined by Feigenbaum (1983).

The term foreman quality control was conceived by Feigenbaum (1983) to denote the quality control of items produced in the early twentieth century (and continuing until approximately 1920) during the Industrial Revolution.

This term was coined to denote the fact that a supervisor or foreman oversaw the quality of goods.

From 1920 to the 1940s, production and processes became more complex, standards were set, and foreman quality control gave way to inspector quality control (Feigenbaum, 1983). In the 1930s, sampling became the norm rather than scrutiny of every single product, in part because this was not feasible during the period of the Second World War. Feigenbaum (1983) labels this period (1930s to 1960s) statistical quality control. Quality control gained attention in England in the 1930s, including the British Standards Institution Standard 600 dealing with applications of statistical methods of quality control (Mitra, 2012). The American Society for Quality Control was formed in 1946, and Japan embraced the notion of statistical quality control with enthusiasm in 1950.

Named again by Feigenbaum (1983), the next phase, total quality control (or total quality management), came into being in the 1960s. At this time, quality control moved away from the inspection department and became the remit of manufacturing departments as manufacturers realized that each department had a role to play in the production of a quality article. At the same time, quality circles gained popularity in Japan (discussed in Chapter 3).

The 1970s saw the advent of the total quality control organization-wide phase, in which all members of the company participated (Feigenbaum, 1983). The total quality system was born in the 1980s (Feigenbaum, 1983).

The 1970s saw the growing use of the cause-and-effect diagram, also known as the Ishikawa diagram (Chapter 3). First introduced in 1946, it began to increase in popularity at this time as a tool to identify possible reasons why a process might become uncontrolled and the likely impacts of this. During the 1970s, Taguchi from Japan introduced the concept of quality improvement through statistically designed experiments (Mitra, 2012).

As computer use increased exponentially in the 1980s, the market was flooded with quality control software. And as the emphasis on customer satisfaction and quality improvement became more important globally, there became a need for a system to support the quality agenda, and so the International Organization for Standardization (ISO) was formed.

The evolution of the information technology era could possibly be described as the most significant development since the Industrial Revolution (Mitra, 2012). The internet has raised expectations in that service providers will be expected to conduct an error-free transaction from production or provision of a service to delivery. According to Mitra, "… the current century will continue to experience a thrust in growth of quality assurance and improvement methods that can, using technology, assimilate data and analyse them in real time and with no tolerance for errors" (2012: 7).

Healthcare organizations

Quality control in healthcare organizations focuses on activities that evaluate, monitor, or regulate services provided to consumers in which processes are observed, characteristics are identified, and variables are tracked through statistical methods (Mitra, 2012).

The following steps should be taken to monitor and evaluate performance in healthcare services:

- Control criteria are established
- Information relevant to the criteria are identified
- The means of collecting information is agreed
- Information is collected and analysed
- The information collected is compared with control criteria
- A judgement is made about quality
- Corrective action is taken if necessary
- Re-evaluate

Total quality management and continuous quality improvement

McLaughlin and Kaluzny (2006) posit that TQM and CQI are one and the same thing, with both terms depicting the planning and execution of a flow of improvement to provide quality care that meets or exceeds expectation. They suggest that TQM and CQI have similar characteristics:

- A link to the organization's strategic plan
- A quality council of staff from the highest level
- Training programmes
- Mechanisms for choosing areas for improvement
- The formation of improvement teams
- Policies that support and motivate staff to take part in improvement processes

Improvements can take place at three levels:

1 *Localized improvements* – when an ad hoc team meets to focus on a particular problem or opportunity
2 *Organizational learning* – the development of policies and procedures, for example protocols or clinical pathways (Chapter 6)
3 *Process re-engineering* – major investment supports the radical amendment to organizational process

McLaughlin and Kaluzny (2006) state that TQM is more likely to be adopted as a part of industry-based programmes, whereas CQI is applied in clinical settings. However, some academics endorse the use of TQM in the delivery of healthcare. Chiarini and Vagnoni (2017) focus on the importance of leadership in the implementation of TQM. They state that TQM has been used in healthcare since the 1980s but not always successfully, which they attribute to the following:

- Lack of senior management involvement and commitment
- Lack of combined leadership in large healthcare organizations
- Lack of political leadership external to healthcare organizations

According to McLaughlin and Kaluzny (2006), CQI comes in a variety of forms but does have a number of essential characteristics:

- Understanding and responding to the organization's external environment
- Empowering clinicians and managers to make improvements
- Acknowledging that customers (patients and providers) are the primary determinants of quality
- Moving away from departmental and professional silos to a multidisciplinary ethos
- Instituting a planned and agreed philosophy of change and adaptation
- Ensuring best practice through organizational learning
- Supporting a rational, data-based approach to analysis and change

Therefore, CQI is both a management philosophy and a management method.

Quality assurance

As described above, quality is no longer the responsibility of one person (operator quality control). In the current age, everyone under the total quality system, or TQM/CQI, is now responsible for quality, whether directly or indirectly. Unfortunately, as has been shown in recent reports (for example, the Francis Report, 2013), something that should be everyone's responsibility becomes no one's responsibility, thus creating an inefficient and ineffective system where quality is paid little more than lip service. Quality assurance is a system whereby all procedures that have been designed and planned are followed (Mitra, 2012). The QA function should continually survey the quality philosophy of the organization, with the quality assurance team auditing all areas to discover and correct errors.

Healthcare organizations

Quality assurance in healthcare should objectively and systematically monitor and evaluate the quality of patient care, improve patient care where possible, and resolve problems as required. The QA process requires a definition of quality, a measurement of quality, and an improvement of quality.

In their article focusing predominantly on the delivery of high-quality care to children, young people, and their families, Corkin and Kenny (2017) examine the challenges and opportunities encountered by children's nurses. With a focus on clinical governance, good communication, teamwork, risk assessment, education, and strong leadership, they examine the challenges of each and suggest ways to delivery patient care of the highest quality. Although focusing specifically on children's nurses in this article, the issues apply to all fields of nursing.

In the UK, a number of policy documents have been published with a view to optimizing standards of care (DHSSPS, 2006; CQC, 2009). However, it is important to remember that the notion of quality of care is likely to have different meanings for different health professionals and the multiple definitions of quality may well lead to a lack of understanding. Furthermore, there is a tension between quality and a cost saving environment. Clinical governance, enforced as it is by various government reports and inquiries in the UK (as discussed in Chapter 1), provides a system of authority whereby the providers of healthcare are accountable.

At a global level, the World Health Organization (2006) states that quality care ought to be:

- Patient-centred
- Equitable
- Accessible
- Effective
- Efficient

Activity 7.1

- How does your workplace address quality issues?
- Which of the above processes are followed (McLaughlin and Kaluzny, 2006)?
- How well are they followed?

Key points

- Quality control is key in clinical governance
- It is widely believed there are four approaches to quality:
  1 QC
  2 TQM
  3 QA
  4 CQI
- McLaughlin and Kaluzny (2006) suggest that TQM and CQI have similar characteristics

---

Clinical risk and risk management

Risk is present in all areas of clinical practice (for example, human error, adverse events, systems failures), and to ameliorate this, risk management is key. Human error, both unpredictable and unintentional, is a rudimentary risk and risk management is essential to identify, assess, and reduce harm to patients, staff, and the public (Clarke and Corkin, 2012). It has been defined as the systematic identification, assessment, and evaluation of risk (Cottee and Harding, 2008). Fenn and Egan argue that not only can risk management be used as an incident-reporting tool, but also "to reduce the risk that clinical or resourcing errors can cause to patients and staff" (2012: 25). Several key reports (for example, Department of Health, 2000, 2004, highlighting the need to learn from clinical errors and improvement to quality of care respectively) have been instrumental in emphasizing the importance and development of risk management.

Risk management is integral to clinical governance. Chandraharan and Arulkumaran (2007) state that clinical governance and risk management form the basis of monitoring patient safety and standards of care. To this end, many elements of risk management are integral to clinical governance, including:

- Risk reporting, including response to complaints
- Audit
- Guidelines
- Risk assessment
- Training

Although not fully up and running until 2000, a risk management programme was implemented in 1995 by the NHS Litigation Authority (NHSLA) (Fenn and Egan, 2012) and Trusts are subject to audit by NHSLA in order to maintain their membership of the Clinical Negligence Scheme for Trusts (CNST). Put simply, risk management encompasses the identification, assessment, and reduction of risks to patients, visitors, staff, and organizational assets.

Any discussion on risk management will inevitably involve a discussion on how to assess risk, as noted above by Chandraharan and Arulkumaran (2007). Clinical risk assessment is complicated, and the three articles discussed below demonstrate the balance that needs to be achieved between risk assessment *per se* and clinical judgement.

As discussed in Chapter 2, pressure ulcers have a significant impact on both patients/carers and organizations. A number of tools have been developed to assess the risk of patients acquiring pressure ulcers, two of the most widely used of which are the Braden Scale and the Norton Scale.

At a micro-level, many speak of the importance of risk assessment tools for pressure ulcers, but Moore and Patton (2019) suggest caution. In 2018, they undertook a search of Cochrane Wounds Specialised Register, the Cochrane Central Register of Controlled Trials (CENTRAL), Ovid MEDLINE (including In-Process & Other Non-Indexed Citations), Ovid Embase, and EBSCO CINAHL Plus. Two eligible studies were included in their review. The first, in which patients were risk-assessed using the Braden Scale, found no discernible difference to patients if clinical judgement alone was used to assess risk. The second study, in which patients were assessed using either the Waterlow or Ramstadius risk assessment tool, produced similar results.

Wei *et al.* (2020) conducted a systematic review to determine the validity and reliability of using the Braden Scale as a risk assessment tool in intensive care units (ICUs). They identified 11 articles with a total sample size of 10,044 patients, 1,058 of whom had pressure ulcers. Their findings showed that the Braden Scale had moderate predictive validity but that either the existing tool needs to be amended or a new tool developed for use in ICUs.

Sullivan, Barnby, and Graham (2020), driven by the fact that no risk assessment scale for pressure ulcers in critical care exists in the USA, undertook a quality improvement project. The aim of their study was to improve the Norton Scale for use with this patient group. The project was based in a 1157-bed academic medical centre in the Southeast United States. Data were collected from 114 clinicians, 111 of whom were critical care nurses; the remaining three were wound care nurses. Using a modified Norton Scale, or optimized Norton Scale (oNS), data were collected on usability, reliability, validity, and preference. The findings showed that the oNS offered a reliable tool that met the above criteria.

As can be seen from the above articles, there appears to be no clear agreement as to the best risk assessment scale for pressure ulcers. This demonstrates that risk assessment can be complicated and highlights the fact that all clinical decisions need to be evidence-based.

An article that appeared in NEJM Catalyst prior to the launch of the *NEJM Catalyst Innovations in Care Delivery* journal (NEJM Catalyst, 2018) discusses the systems and processes used to identify and mitigate risk in healthcare settings. There it is stated that advances in the delivery of healthcare, such as new healthcare technologies and cybersecurity technologies, and changes to the regulatory, legal, and political agendas regularly impact on risk management, making it more complex than it was previously. The article suggests eight risk domains:

- Operational
- Clinical/patient safety
- Strategic
- Financial
- Human capital
- Legal/regulatory
- Technology
- Hazard

Furthermore, it is suggested that risk managers involve staff and patients to help them identify risks. It is important to remember that this is not a single assessment of risk but an ongoing process. Risk management involves the identification of past and current patient care incidents and other events that may present a potential loss to the organization (Kavaler and Spiegel, 2003).

The identification of possible liability risks such as unexpected treatment outcomes, complaints, and adverse events must be an ongoing process. Research shows that more often than not, safety failures are due to poorly designed management systems, suggesting that organizational failures are more prevalent than individual failures (Currie and Watterson, 2007). This being the case, individuals managing teams and/or budgets must ensure that the service delivered is safe and effective.

Teamwork is essential in preventing organizational failures. Not only does it support a shared vision, but it also increases awareness of the clinical expertise that each team member brings. Integrated care is best achieved by an interdisciplinary approach (Corkin and Kenny, 2017) where efficient communication is key.

Additionally, transformational nurse leaders, and we have discussed the importance of leadership throughout this book, are able to influence guidelines, motivate teams, and encourage team members to support one another in a non-threatening environment. Some authors (Armitage, Newell, and Wright, 2010) consider frontline healthcare staff as being at the sharp end and managers at the blunt end. Such discrimination sometimes leads to frontline staff being unaware of the bigger picture and therefore somewhat resistant to change. Despite efforts to the contrary, there is still a culture of blame within health services (Corkin and Kenny, 2017), and negative experiences and bullying will prevent nurses from challenging unsafe practices.

Corkin and Kenny (2017) suggest the following:

- Quantify and prioritize risk – once identified, risks should be scored and prioritized based on likelihood of occurrence and impact
- Investigate and report Sentinel Events
- Capture and learn from near misses – these should be reported as they often help to identify risk and are fundamental to risk assessment and management
- Think beyond the obvious to identify latent failures – for example, a medication error is an easily identified error. A latent failure, for example, is where poor lighting might have made it difficult to read the patient's chart and therefore led to the error. It is important to consider underlying and less obvious causes
- Use models, for example root cause analysis, to understand obvious and latent failures
- Invest in a risk management information system
- Find a balance between risk financing and risk transfer, for example insurance policies. Risk financing requires an understanding and evaluation of the finances involved, such as insurance and liability costs

In the USA, the American Society of Healthcare Risk Management (ASHRM) offers a risk management programme (Kavaler and Spiegel, 2003) in which:

- There will be a designated risk manager who will receive at least eight hours of risk management training annually
- Risk managers will have access to all data, whether medical or management
- A written policy statement regarding risk management will be agreed by the governing body, the medical staff, and administration of the organization
- There will be a system to identify, review, and analyse all adverse outcomes, unanticipated or otherwise
- Risk management data will be centralized
- A report from the risk manager will be presented annually to the governing body of the organization
- Risk managers will ensure that all medical staff and new employees attend educational programmes on minimizing clinical risk and high-risk clinical areas
- Risk managers are required to forward all information on malpractice and adverse outcomes to the committees that evaluate the competence of medical staff

The report also strongly suggests that healthcare organizations need a risk management plan to guide how the organization identifies, manages, and mitigates risk. Risk management plans are likely to vary from organization to organization, but key to all plans are:

- Education and training such as ongoing and in-service training
- Patient and family grievances/complaints to promote patient satisfaction. Grievances/complaints should be documented including response times, staff responsibilities, and action taken
- Purpose, goals, and metrics to reduce Sentinel Events, near misses, and liability claims. The plan should also require regular reporting systems to be in place
- A communication plan to promote open dialogue and a no blame culture
- Contingency plans for adverse system-wide failures such as security breaches, long-term power loss, or disease outbreaks
- Reporting protocols which are quick and easy to use
- Response and mitigation plans to respond to reported risks and lessons learnt

Risk control or treatment

This is the organization's response to significant risk areas and is the most common function of risk management programmes. Kavaler and Spiegel (2003) list a combination of techniques for controlling risk:

1 *Risk acceptance* – the organization takes a measured decision not to purchase insurance against a particular adverse event

2 *Exposure avoidance* – removing the service, personnel, or equipment that may cause the loss

3 *Loss prevention* – improving education for staff; improving communication with patients when a mishap occurs in the hope that this will produce a satisfied patient who will not sue the organization

4 *Loss reduction* – education, revision of policies and procedures

5 *Exposure segregation* – separate out the "offending" service, for example in the case of medication errors, all drugs can be dispensed from a central location

6 *Contractual transfer* – contract the service out to another provider

---

Activity 7.2

Think about when TGN1412 was used in a clinical trial in 2006 and six young men went into organ failure hours after taking the drug. How might the six points above impact on further drug trials?

Whilst drug trials such as TGN1412 are essential in the acceptance of new treatments, organizations managing these trials have to control the risk. They have a responsibility to ensure that risk is mitigated through treatment of potential side effects and have to ensure that finances are available for compensation.

Risk management tools

The following tools may be used to identify risk:

- *Incident reporting* – report incidents such as when a patient falls while trying to get into bed
- *Occurrence reporting* – some insurers require organizations to develop a list of adverse patient occurrences that are to be reported by staff, for example, maternal or infant death, the unplanned return of a surgical patient to the hospital, or an allergic reaction to medication
- *Occurrence screening* – these identify occurrences that are at variance with normal practice, for example the transfer of a patent from a general ward to ICU, nosocomial infections, or an unanticipated return to theatre

The link between risk management and quality assurance

Risk management and quality assurance are two activities that sometimes overlap (Kavaler and Spiegel, 2003), as shown in Tables 7.1 and 7.2.

Table 7.1 Similarities between risk management and quality assurance

Risk management	Quality assurance
Protects the financial assets of the institution	Demonstrates the organization's caring philosophy
Protects humans and resources	Improves the performance of all staff
Protects humans and property	and protects patients
Reduces loss by focusing on individual loss or accidents	Focuses on the delivery of quality care
	According to standards and measurable
Prevents incidents by improving quality of care through monitoring of activities	criteria, sets quality of care requirement
	Continuously monitors problem areas to prevent future incidents
Examines each incident using the risk management process:	Searches for non-conformance using quality assurance processes:
• Risk identification	• Problem identification
• Risk analysis	• Problem assessment
• Risk control	• Corrective action
• Risk financing	• Follow-up
	• Report of findings

Table 7.2 Differences between risk management and quality assurance

Risk management	Quality assurance
Concerned with acceptable levels of care from a legal view	Concerned with best level of care
Focuses on all humans and events	Focuses on patient care
Focuses on legal, insurance, and risk financing activities	Focuses on improving care

Carroll (2009), in her edited text on healthcare risk management, cites the following steps as essential to the risk management process:

• Identify and analyse loss exposure, for example property, liability, personnel
• Consider alternative risk techniques, for example exposure avoidance, loss reduction, segregation of exposure, contractual transfer
• Select the best risk single or combination of management techniques
• Implement
• Monitor (evaluate) and improve the risk management programme

As can be seen, Carroll (2009) includes areas very similar to those of Kavaler and Spiegel (2003), but she includes evaluation as a key element of risk management.

Key points

- Risk management and quality assurance are different, although some overlap is evident
- Risk management focuses on financial management
- Quality assurance focuses on quality of care

Tom Hellmich, physician and Minneapolis Children's Hospital Patient Safety Council member, states in the *Risk Management Handbook for Healthcare Organisations* that the "medical culture that silently taught the ABCs as Accuse, Blame, and Criticize is fading. Rising in its place is a safety culture emphasizing blameless reporting, successful systems, knowledge, respect, confidentiality, and trust" (NEJM Catalyst, 2018).

Complaints management

As mentioned in Chapter 6, clinical negligence costs represent a major threat to the viability of the NHS, which paid £2.4bn (€2.8bn; $3.1bn) in clinical negligence claims in 2018–2019 according to NHS Resolution (2020) (formerly the NHS Litigation Authority). This sum equals approximately 2% of the NHS budget in England (Office of National Statistics, 2019). Abdelrahman and Abdelmageed (2017) attribute complaints to concerns about investigations and treatments, a breakdown in communication, and lack of respect for the patient.

McSherry and Pearce (2011) state that the vast majority of claims are resolved locally, stressing that openness and honesty, together with robust systems to deal with issues before they become problems, are the main ways of dealing with complaints. Organizations need to develop a learning culture that supports employees to report, discuss, and learn from incidents, and McSherry and Pearce stress that often complaints arise from systems failure rather than the action of a single member of staff.

McSherry and Pearce (2011) present a case study in which a Trust has received a number of complaints from patients (and their carers) who have been admitted to the medical ward following a stroke. The complaints can be divided into poor quality care and poor communication and are illustrated in Table 7.3.

A clinical governance framework supports the organization in understanding and responding to the problem that is distressing patients and carers. In the case outlined above, the process might be:

- Clinical risk identified by letters of complaint, letters acknowledged and investigated by the complaints manager
- Poor quality care identified (poor patient care and poor communication, as above)
- Review of systems and processes required

Table 7.3 Analysis of complaints

Poor quality care	Poor communication
• Poor attendance to privacy and hygiene needs • Development of pressure sores • Poor attention to nutritional needs • Limited access to physiotherapy, occupational health, and rehabilitation • Home assessment and discharge delayed	• Limited information to patient and carers • Inconsistent information from healthcare staff • Failure to disclose information about patient falls • Inadequate capture of patient safety data

- Clinical audit carried out to explore the nature of the complaint
- Review of the literature carried out to understand best practice
- Audit of current process against best practice, identified in point 5 above relating to the risk management process (this may lead to the need for education and training; Chapter 5), and recommendations made, implemented, and re-audited within 12 months)
- Review of patient outcomes
- Leading to a reduction in complaints and a general increase in satisfaction levels

In the case study given by McSherry and Pearce (2011), the complaints were related to poor systems and processes with which the clinicians had to work, rather than to the clinicians themselves. Following the process above would encourage a review of best evidence-based practice against which changes to practice could be made. This would also enable the organization to learn from any mistakes.

The Patients Association, an independent charity campaigning on improvements in health and social care, issued a report (2013) into complaint handling in NHS Trusts that are signed up to the CARE (2011) campaign. The CARE campaign was launched in 2011 and focuses on the four most common complaints notified to their helpline:

- Poor communication
- Poor attention to toileting needs
- Poor attention to nutritional needs
- Pain relief

The Complaints Regulations for England (Local Authority Social Services and National Health Service Complaints [England] Regulations, 2009) and Wales (National Health Service Concerns, Complaints and Redress Arrangements [Wales] Regulations, 2011) require all Trusts to have systems in place to "ensure effective, timely and consistent management of complaints" and courteous and respectful treatment of complaints. The Care Quality Commission standards of quality and safety and the Ombudsman's principles of good complaint handling also support NHS organizations in the management of complaints. The Patients Association's report listed 10 criteria that identified good practice in the complaints handling system of the 20 randomly selected Trusts who took part in their research. These are as follows:

- *Criterion 1*: A responsible person. Under the Complaints Regulations for England and Wales there is a requirement for a senior member of staff to take overall responsibility for the management of complaints. This person will be responsible for the complaints management team and a governance committee, both of which will report to the Trust board regularly
- *Criterion 2*: An exhaustive complaints policy. The Patients Association suggests that the complaints policy of all Trusts should be visible on their websites
- *Criterion 3*: An explanation of the complaints policy in plain language, either on a website or via leaflets
- *Criteria 4 and 5*: Regular reporting to the Trust board
- *Criterion 6*: Production and publication of regular complaints reports, ideally on the Trust website
- *Criterion 7*: Production of annual reports and quality accounts – ideally to be produced by all Trusts
- *Criterion 8*: Staff training – this should also include policy documents on complaints management
- *Criteria 9 and 10*: A culture of and provision for active learning from complaints – this needs to be well developed and at all levels of the organization

It is interesting to compare these 10 criteria with the findings of the Healthwatch report (2020), which is discussed later in this chapter.

Overview of the main complaints regulations in England and Wales

The NHS Constitution (2013), which lists the rights and responsibilities of staff and patients, sets out some key principles to guide the NHS. Among these are:

- The provision of a comprehensive service to all, based on clinical need rather than ability to pay
- A commitment to taxpayers, ensuring good value for money
- To be accountable to patients, communities, and the public
- To aspire to the highest standards of professionalism and excellence

In other words, the provision of care that is safe, effective, and focused on the experience of the patient.

All NHS, private, and third sector providers are legally required to adopt the NHS Constitution in all their dealings with patients, and the rights of complaint and redress are encompassed within this. The Constitution makes the following explicit statements:

- The right to have any complaint you make about NHS services dealt with efficiently and to have it properly investigated
- The right to know the outcome of any investigation into your complaint
- The right to take your complaint to the independent Health Service Ombudsman, if you are not satisfied with the way your complaint has been dealt with by the NHS

An updated version of the NHS Constitution (2021), available on the gov.uk website, gives further detail on what patients/carers should expect when making a complaint:

- Their complaint, whether made verbally, in writing, or electronically, will be acknowledged within three working days. The exception to this is where an oral complaint is resolved no later than the next day
- They will be offered the opportunity to discuss how their complaint will be handled
- They will be informed of the timeframe of when the complaint will be investigated and when they will receive a response
- The response will detail the conclusions of the investigation and what actions will be taken as a result of the complaint

Normally, complaints must be made within 12 months of an issue occurring or within 12 months of the complainant becoming aware that there is an issue. The 2009 regulations also stipulate the requirement for the publicity, monitoring, and reporting of complaints (Local Authority Social Services and National Health Service Complaints [England] Regulations, 2009), stating that arrangements for dealing with complaints and how those arrangements may be obtained.

According to the Health and Social Care Act (2012), NHS organizations not only have a legal obligation but also have a contractual obligation and have to be registered with the Care Quality Commission, who will ensure that the provision of care meets set standards of quality and safety (CQC, 2010). The CQC give 28 outcomes, 16 of which specifically relate to quality and safety of care, clearly stating that each registered body must:

- Have systems in place to deal with comments and complaints
- Support patients/carers to make comments and complaints
- Consider, respond to, and resolve all comments and complaints where possible

The Parliamentary and Health Service Ombudsman

When a complaint is not resolved locally, it will be directed to the Parliamentary and Health Service Ombudsman for further investigation following the principles described in their Principles of Good Complaint Handling (Parliamentary and Health Service Ombudsman, 2009). These are as follows:

- Getting it right
- Being customer-focused
- Being open and accountable
- Acting fairly and proportionately
- Putting things right
- Seeking continuous improvement

However, a review in late 2012 (Parliamentary and Health Service Ombudsman, 2012) of complaint handling in England showed an 8% rise in complaints, highlighting communication problems with complainants. In the period between 2010/11 and 2011/12, the Ombudsman highlighted 50% more complaints about the NHS not acknowledging mistakes in care, 13% more complaints about the NHS providing poor explanations to complainants, and 42% more complaints about inadequate resolutions.

***

Activity 7.3

- The paragraphs above focus on systems in the UK. How does your country/healthcare provider deal with complaints if you do not work in the UK?
- What happens at the local level?
- If not resolved at the local level, how are these complaints resolved?

***

Serious failings and lessons learnt

We have previously discussed the Mid Staffordshire NHS Foundation Trust, where governance and operational failings of more than a decade resulted in high mortality and complaints were ignored. It was the Healthcare Commission that, in March 2009, highlighted the problems in their investigation into the Trust's high mortality rates for patients admitted as emergencies (Healthcare Commission, 2009). Many issues were uncovered, including complaints not being presented to the Trust board appropriately, and a lack of openness to encourage the discussion and consequent resolution of complaints. The Healthcare Commission (2009: 11–12) proposed the following regarding future practice in Trusts:

> Trusts to ensure that systems for governance that appear to be persuasive on paper actually work in practice, and information presented to Boards on performance (including complaints and incidents) is not so summarized that it fails to convey the experience of patients or enable non-executives to scrutinize and challenge on issues relating to patients' care.

Furthermore, the Commission charged Mid Staffordshire to improve its quality of care by:

- Developing and supporting an open learning culture

- Collecting accurate information and reporting it appropriately
- Investigating and learning from serious incidents such as unexpected deaths
- Ensuring improvements are made following near misses, incidents, and complaints
- Identifying and reducing risks
- Engaging clinicians and developing effective clinical audit
- Listening to patients

These recommendations should be implemented in all healthcare organizations, thereby supporting a strong complaints system, as they echo the Health Service Ombudsman's principles of good complaint handling.

The Healthcare Commission's inquiry prompted an independent inquiry, chaired by Sir Robert Francis QC, and the inquiry reported in February 2010, revealing neglect and systems failings (including patient experience, staff perceptions, and the culture of the Trust) at Mid Staffordshire NHS Foundation Trust. Complaints were supposedly channelled to the board through the Medical Director and Director of Nursing only, but there was little or no evidence of complaints reaching the chief executive or the board. Rather, the investigation of complaints was predominantly handled at a very local level, that is, staff in the area of the complaint, resulting in defensiveness rather than constructive reporting and learning. The reporting of complaints was slow and did not always address all the issues raised, nor was remedial action implemented. The Francis Inquiry team concluded that a "poor complaints system has a negative impact on patents and others who seek to use it. Inadequate responses cause distress and may exacerbate bereavement" (Francis Report, 2013: 20).

The Francis Inquiry advised the Mid Staffordshire Trust board to:

- Ensure adequate responses and plans for resolution of complaints
- Ensure that staff are engaged at all levels of the process, that is, from investigation to implementation of lessons learnt
- Minimize the risk of the problem occurring again
- Make information on complaints and their resolution available to the board, the governors, and the public

Furthermore, these recommendations would be useful to all Trusts, and, in fact, Recommendation 18 of the Francis Report is: "All NHS trusts and foundation trusts responsible for the provision of hospital services should review their standards, governance and performance in the light of this report" (2013: 28).

Nearly seven years later, in January 2020, Healthwatch, an independent service for users of health and social care, produced a document about patient complaints. The foreword to the document was written by Sir Robert Francis QC. In his final report of the Mid Staffordshire inquiry, he stated that the processes whereby complaints are handled should ensure that outcomes are shared with the public in order to prevent similar serious failures in the future. Many of the recommendations made in the report have been implemented, for example NHS Digital now publishes quarterly complaints reports including theme, provider, and service area. Despite these advances, however, a survey undertaken by the Care Quality Commission (2019) found that almost 7 million people who accessed health or social care services in the previous five years had concerns about their care but did not raise them. Those who did raise concerns have seen an improvement to the service. Francis stated that it is imperative that patients who have concerns must raise them, and the NHS must respond by showing those patients the direct improvements that occur as a result. It continues to be hard for members of the public who make complaints to see the positive impact their complaint has had on the system as a whole.

The Healthwatch report (2020) investigated how well NHS hospital Trusts across England conveyed information on complaints and whether this was sufficient to build public confidence in the process. They searched the websites of 149 NHS acute Trusts in England to examine their reporting procedures. They found that:

- Local reporting on complaints was inconsistent and inaccessible with only 12% of hospital Trusts compliant with statutory regulations
- Staff were not empowered to communicate with the public about complaints
- Reporting focused on counting complaints rather than demonstrating learning – for example, only 38% of Trusts demonstrated what changes they had made in response to complaints

Furthermore, Healthwatch found that only 44% of Trusts included useful information in their annual reports about the types of complaints they received and how they dealt with them. Additionally, Trusts are legally required to make their reports available to anyone on request, but this seems not be have been the case when Healthwatch contacted 15 Trusts with a request to access their annual complaints reports. Only four provided them with the information they had requested.

The Healthwatch report (2020) asks a number of pertinent questions:

- How are hospitals reporting on complaints?
- How easy is it to access reports on request?
- Are Trusts complying with complaints regulations?
- How transparent are Trusts in their reporting of complaints?
- How well do Trusts demonstrate what they have learnt from the complaints they receive?
- How well do Trusts think they learn from complaints?
- Is the language of complaints causing confusion as to how Trusts report complaints?
- Should formal and informal complaints be recorded in the same way?
- Are third party complaints recorded?

It also makes a number of recommendations:

- There is a need to improve transparency, particularly in how leaning from complaints is communicated to the public in order to improve public confidence
- Managers and staff should be empowered to demonstrate learning from complaints
- There should be a system-wide approach whereby a national complaints standards authority is tasked with developing best practice, training, and monitoring of reporting and learning from complaints

It is good to see that a number of improvements have been made to the complaints process since the failures noted at Mid Staffordshire NHS Foundation Trust. However, it is concerning that the system does not appear to be robust enough to prevent such failures from ever occurring again.

Summary

From the above it can be seen that best practice of the management of complaints should include the following:

- Openness – Trusts must be open and accountable to the public and complaints must be handled thoroughly and transparently
- Trusts must have an up-to-date complaints policy, clearly outlining responsibilities, the steps in the complaints handling procedure, and the mechanisms used to report to the Trust board, for example via the annual report, the complaints report, etc.
- The complaints system must be clearly stated on the Trust's website and given in plain English. Leaflets can supplement the use of a website
- All complaints must be reported to the Trust board at each Trust board meeting, and all documents discussed during the public part of the board meeting must be available on the website. Additionally, complaints data and trends must be discussed at every board meeting
- Trusts must produce complaints reports (including at the least, statistics, trend analysis, lessons learned, and actions taken) and these must be published on their website
- Trusts must make public their annual reports and quality accounts every year
- Trusts must invest in staff training in the handling of complaints so that staff are cognisant of the complaints-handling regulations and mechanisms
- All complaints must be taken seriously, reported, and investigated so that incidents do not re-occur
- Trusts must support an open learning culture. Lessons must be learned following a complaint, and complainants must receive a letter detailing what

action the Trust has taken together with a later update on the action. Each annual teport, quality account, and complaints report must include a section on actions taken and lessons learned. All improvements need to be publicized widely

Additionally, the Patients Association, in their report *Complaint Handling in NHS Trusts* (2013), signed up to the CARE campaign, and made the following recommendations, which mirror those above:

- All NHS Trusts must be able to demonstrate that they follow all regulations, obligations, and recommendations related to complaints. Trusts without a clear complaints policy must develop one
- All NHS Trusts must be able to demonstrate openness, accountability, and transparency in relation to complaints
- All NHS Trusts must listen to patients and show respect and understanding rather than defensiveness
- Many complaints are due to poor communication. Patients' rights and choices with regard to complaints must be well communicated to them, their carers, and their families
- The NHS Constitution must be published on all Trust websites as well as on posters throughout the Trust
- Information on how to make a complaint must be available on the Trust website, as well as on posters and in leaflets in the wards and treatment areas
- Complaints reports presented at board meetings must be made available on the Trust website
- Complaint-related staff training needs to be identified and made available for all relevant staff
- Improvements made after complaints or incidents must be publicized
- Best practice is to be understood, agreed, and consistently applied to the Trust's complaints system

---

Key points

- All NHS, private, and third sector providers are legally required to adopt the NHS Constitution in all of their dealings with patients
- The rights of complaint and redress are encompassed within the NHS Constitution
- Empowering patients/service users and staff to enable them to shape governance strategies collaboratively (shared governance) will reduce complaints

Empowering patients/service users and staff to enable them to shape governance strategies collaboratively

Definitions of shared governance are somewhat confusing. Hess (2004) describes it as follows: "Shared governance is a journey, not a destination. Organisations pursuing shared governance move incrementally from past orientations where the few rule to an orientation where many learn to make consensual decisions". Hess goes on to state that "nursing shared governance is hard to define. Its structures and processes are different in every organisation".

Porter-O'Grady possibly gives a more helpful definition: "Shared governance is, in short, simply a structural model through which nurses can express and manage their practice with a higher level of professional autonomy" (2004: 251).

The literature suggests that the common characteristics of shared governance include accountability, empowerment, participation, and collaboration in decisions that affect patient care, including decisions once held to be the realm of management.

Nurses who are involved in shared governance need to be orientated towards constant change and professional development and also acknowledge the need for a cultural shift in their organization. Additionally, and importantly, Hess (2004) argues that shared governance should include everyone's voice, including that of patients: "Shared governance models that include only nurses can become exclusionary and eventually ineffectual by focusing on the goals of a single profession, instead of the organisation as a whole".

There is increasingly more literature highlighting how patients are included in decision-making, supporting the concept of patients becoming co-designers (as discussed in Chapter 1) of the delivery of their treatment. Shared decision-making that includes the patient's voice has been associated with improved health outcomes and high patient satisfaction (Edward and Elwyn, 2009).

Stigglebout *et al.* (2012) argue that the most important reason for supporting patients to engage in shared decision-making is one of ethics. Beauchamp and Childress (2001) present three ethical principles that should be applied to shared decision-making:

1 Supporting patients to make reasoned informed choices supports their autonomy

2 Supporting patients to make reasoned informed choices supports the concept of beneficence by balancing the benefits of treatment against risks and cost, and therefore non-maleficence (avoiding harm)

3 Supporting patients to make reasoned informed choices supports the concept of justice (distributing benefits, risks, and costs fairly) as patients usually make more conservative decisions than doctors, and often elect to have fewer procedures

However, despite these benefits, shared decision-making is far from routine. Stigglebout *et al.* (2012) suggest the need for a position of equipoise or balance, suggesting to the patient that there is often no best choice, that a decision must be made, and that doing nothing is also an option. Patients must be given all the facts and will need statistics to weigh up the pros and cons.

In the past, it has been argued, most decision-making was made by well-educated middle-class patients in high-income countries. However, evidence now suggests that providing information in a way that is accessible to patients with lower literacy levels enables them to make informed decisions about their care.

Whatever the aspired goal, shared decision-making requires a cultural shift among healthcare professionals, organizations, and patients, but the ultimate goal must be that patients are at the centre of all decisions pertaining to their health. This is encapsulated in the Salzburg Statement on Shared Decision-Making (2011), which calls on clinicians to:

- Acknowledge that they have an ethical obligation to share important decisions with patients
- Motivate two-way communication, which not only gives information but encourages patients to ask questions and thereby offer their preferred method of treatment
- Provide accurate information about options, uncertainties, benefits, and harms of the treatment options

Barry and Edgman-Levitan (2012) present eight characteristics of care from the perspective of patients:

1 Respect for the patient's values, preferences, and expressed needs
2 Coordinated and integrated care
3 Clear, high-quality information and education for patients, their carers, and families
4 Physical comfort, including pain management
5 Emotional support and a reduction of fear and anxiety
6 Involvement of carers, families, and friends
7 Continuity of care
8 Access to care

All of these are possible if patients and their families are empowered to design, implement, and evaluate care systems.

More recent research endorses the importance of involving patients in the co-design of their healthcare. Using focus groups and interviews, Williams, Turner, and Beadle (2018) undertook a qualitative study in the UK to examine the views of patients attending a pulmonary rehabilitation (PR) programme. Three focus groups were held involving 33 patients. Additionally, semi-structured interviews were carried out with 15 patients. The authors' findings demonstrated the benefits and challenges to patients attending a PR programme and, as a result, a patient-led redesign group was initiated to improve the programme, thus ensuring that it continued to meet patient needs. Additionally, it was agreed that focus groups would be held annually to ensure that the patients' voice remained central to the ongoing development and redesign of the programme, with quality improvement projects ensuring that this is the case.

Furthermore, Goodrich (2018) states that, as patients have first-hand knowledge of their care from start to finish, they should be included in the design or redesign of services.

Clarke *et al.* (2017), in the first systematic review to investigate outcomes associated with developing and implementing co-designed healthcare interventions, found that reported outcomes related to:

- The value of co-designed processes
- The generation of ideas for change to healthcare delivery
- Concrete service changes and their impact on patients

Whilst these are important points, they felt that little regard had been given to evaluating the sustainability of changes made, a cost analysis of changes made, or an economic evaluation. It is unclear from the articles discussed above whether these points had been taken into account.

Activity 7.4

- Thinking about your place of work, how well are patients supported in making decisions about their treatment?
- Who blocks this process and why?
- How might you be able to support your patients in becoming more autonomous?

Key point

Patients should be involved in the design, implementation, and evaluation of healthcare systems (co-designing – Chapter 1).

Key points summary

There are four approaches to quality: quality control, total quality management, quality assurance, and continuous quality improvement. Quality control evaluates, monitors, and regulates services provided to consumers. TQM and CQI differ from one another but do have some similarities:

- TQM and CQI both link to the organization's strategic plan, involve education and training, and focus on areas for improvement
- CQI is more likely to refer to the clinical setting, whereas TQM is more industry-based

CQI is a management philosophy and is central to clinical governance. Risk management involves risk identification, risk analysis, risk control, and risk financing. Risk management focuses on finances, whereas quality assurance focuses on care, but there are also similarities:

- Both protect the service user
- They both prevent incidents by continuously monitoring activities

The four most common complaints are poor communication, poor attention to toileting needs, poor attention to nutritional needs, and poor pain relief. These complaints can be reduced by empowering patients/service users and staff through shared governance (accountability, empowerment, participation, and collaboration).

Implications for practice

- It is imperative that staff report "near misses", as these inform risk management
- Teams/staff should be involved in risk analysis, so that they understand what happened and why it happened
- All staff need to know how to access the complaints procedure
- If possible, complaints should first be sensitively dealt with at the local level
- All staff need to be cognisant of the organization's policies pertaining to complaints that cannot be resolved at the local level

End-of-chapter questions

1 What is the key difference between quality assurance and CQI?
2 What is the difference between quality assurance and risk management?
3 How does a poor complaints system impact on patients, carers, and staff?

See the Appendix on page 256 for suggested answers to these questions.

References

Abdelrahman, W. and Abdelmageed, A. (2017) Understanding patient complaints, *British Medical Journal*, 356: j452. Available at: https://doi.org/10.1136/bmj.j452.

Armitage, G., Newell, R., and Wright, J. (2010) Improving the quality of medication error reporting, *Journal of Evaluation in Clinical Practice*, 16 (6): 1189–1197.

Barry, M.J. and Edgman-Levitan, S. (2012) Shared decision-making: The pinnacle of patient-centred care, *New England Journal of Medicine*, 366 (9): 780–781.

Beauchamp, T.L. and Childress, J.F. (2001) *Principles of Biomedical Ethics*, 5th edition. Oxford: Oxford University Press.

CARE Campaign (2011) Available at: http:/www.thecarecampaign.co.uk/ (accessed: 7 March 2021).

Care Quality Commission (CQC) (2009) *Guidance on Compliance: Essential standards of quality and safety.* Available at: www.cqc.org.uk/guidance-providers/regulations-enforcement/about-guidance (accessed: 7 March 2021).

Care Quality Commission (CQC) (2010) *Guidance about compliance: Summary of regulations, outcomes and judgement framework.* Available at: https://minhalexander.files.wordpress.com/2018/08/cqc-2010-guidance_about_compliance_summary.pdf (accessed: 7 March 2021).

Care Quality Commission (CQC) (2019) *New research for CQC shows people regret not raising concerns about their care – but those who do raise concerns see improvements*, Press release, 19 February. Available at: https://www.cqc.org.uk/news/releases/new-research-cqc-shows-people-regret-not-raising-concerns-about-their-care-those-who (accessed: 7 March 2021).

Carroll, R. (2009) *Risk Management Handbook for Healthcare Organizations.* San Francisco, CA: Jossey-Bass.

Chandraharan, E. and Arulkumaran, S. (2007) Clinical governance, *Obstetrics, Gynaecology and Reproductive Medicine*, 17 (7): 222–224.

Chiarini, A. and Vagnoni, E. (2017) TQI implementation for the healthcare sector: The relevance of leadership and possible causes of lack of leadership, *Leadership in Health Services*, 30 (3): 210–216.

Clarke, D., Jones, F., Harris, R., and Robert, G. (2017) What outcomes are associated with developing and implementing co-produced interventions in acute healthcare settings? A rapid evidence synthesis, *BMJ Open*, 7: e014650. Available at: https://doi.org/10.1136/bmjopen-2016-014650.

Clarke, S. and Corkin, D. (2012) Risk assessment and management, in D. Corkin, S. Clarke, and L. Liggett (eds.) *Care Planning in Children and Young People's Nursing.* Chichester: Wiley-Blackwell.

Corkin, D. and Kenny, J. (2017) Quality patient care: Challenges and opportunities, *Nursing Management*, 24 (7): 32–36.

Cottee, C. and Harding, K. (2008) Risk management in obstetrics, *Obstetrics, Gynaecology and Reproductive Medicine*, 18: 155–162.

Currie, L. and Watterson, L. (2007) Challenges in delivering safe patient care: A commentary on a quality improvement initiative, *Journal of Nursing Management*, 15 (2): 162–168.

Department of Health (2000) *An Organisation with a Memory.* London: Department of Health.

Department of Health (2004) *National Standards, Local Action: The health and social care standards and planning framework 2005/6–2007/8.* Available at: https://webarchive.nationalarchives.gov.uk/20081211193841/http://www.dh.gov.uk/en/Publicationsandstatistics/Publications/PublicationsPolicyAndGuidance/DH_4086057 (accessed: 25 June 2021).

Department of Health, Social Services, and Public Safety (DHSSPS) (2006) *Quality Standards for Health and Social Care*. Belfast: DHSSPS.

Edward, A. and Elwyn, G. (eds.) (2009) *Shared Decision-Making in Healthcare: Achieving evidence-based patient choice*, 2nd edition. Oxford: Oxford University Press.

Feigenbaum, A.V. (1983) *Total Quality Control*. New York: McGraw-Hill.

Fenn, P. and Egan, T. (2012) Risk management in the NHS: Governance, finance and clinical risk, *Clinical Medicine*, 12 (1): 25–28.

Francis Report (2013) *Report of the Mid Staffordshire NHS Trust Foundation Trust Public Inquiry*. London: HMSO.

Goodrich, J. (2018) Why experience-based co-design improves the patient experience, *Journal of Health Design*, 3 (1): 84–85.

Health and Social Care Act (2012) Available at: https://www.legislation.gov.uk/ukpga/2012/7/contents/enacted (accessed: 7 March 2021).

Healthcare Commission (2009) *Investigation into Mid Staffordshire NHS Foundation Trust*. Available at: https://www.bl.uk/collection-items/investigation-into-mid-staffordshire-nhs-foundation-trust# (accessed: 7 March 2021).

Healthwatch (2020) *Shifting the Mindset: A closer look at hospital complaints*. Available at: https://www.healthwatch.co.uk/sites/healthwatch.co.uk/files/20191126%20-%20 Shifting%20the%20mindset%20-%20NHS%20complaints%20.pdf (accessed: 7 March 2021).

Hess, R.G. (2004) From bedside to boardroom – nursing shared governance, *Online Journal of Issues in Nursing*, 9 (1). Available at: https://ojin.nursingworld.org/Main-MenuCategories/ANAMarketplace/ANAPeriodicals/OJIN/TableofContents/Volume92004/No1Jan04/FromBedsidetoBoardroom.html (accessed: 7 March 2021).

Kavaler, F. and Spiegel, A. (2003) *Risk Management in Healthcare Institutions: A strategic approach*, 2nd edition. Mississauga, ON: Jones & Bartlett.

Local Authority Social Services and National Health Service Complaints (England) Regulations (2009). Available at: http://www.legislation.gov.uk/uksi/2009/309/regulation/4/made (accessed: 7 March 2021).

McLaughlin, C.P. and Kaluzny, A.D. (2006) *Continuous Quality Improvement in Healthcare: Theory, implementations and applications*, 3rd edition. London: Jones & Bartlett.

McSherry, R. and Pearce, P. (2011) *Clinical Governance: A guide to implementation for healthcare professionals*, 3rd edition. Oxford: Wiley-Blackwell.

Mitra, A. (2012) *Fundamentals of Quality Control and Improvement*. Hoboken, NJ: Wiley.

Moore, Z.E.H. and Patton, D. (2019) Risk assessment tools for the prevention of pressure ulcers. *Cochrane Database of Systematic Reviews*, 1: CD006471. Available at: https://doi.org/10.1002/14651858.CD006471.pub4.

National Health Service (Concerns, Complaints and Redress Arrangements) (Wales), Regulations (2011) Available a: http://www.legislation.gov.uk/wsi/2011/704/pdfs/wsi_20110704_mi.pdf (accessed: 7 March 2021).

NEJM Catalyst (2018) *What is Risk Management in Healthcare?* Available at: https://catalyst.nejm.org/doi/full/10.1056/CAT.18.0197 (accessed: 7 March 2021).

NHS Constitution (2013) Available at: http://www.england.nhs.uk/2013/03/26/nhs-constitution/ (accessed: 7 March 2021).

NHS Constitution (2021) *NHS Complaints Guidance*. Available at: https://www.gov.uk/government/publications/the-nhs-constitution-for-england/how-do-i-give-feedback-or-make-a-complaint-about-an-nhs-service#giving-feedback (accessed: 7 March 2021).

NHS Resolution (2020) *Annual Report and Accounts 2019/20*. Available at: https://resolution.nhs.uk/2020/07/16/nhs-resolutions-annual-report-and-accounts-2019-20/ (accessed: 25 June 2021).

Office of National Statistics (ONS) (2019) Available at: https://www.ons.gov.uk/search-publication?q=complaints%20NHS (accessed: 7 March 2021).

Parliamentary and Health Service Ombudsman (2009) *Principles of Good Complaint Handling*. Available at: http://www.ombudsman.org.uk/improving-public-service/ombudsmansprinciples/principles-of-good-complaint-handling-full (accessed: 7 March 2021).

Parliamentary and Health Service Ombudsman (2012) *Listening and Learning: The Ombudsman's review of complaint handling in the NHS in England 2011–12*. Available at: https://www.ombudsman.org.uk/publications/listening-and-learning-ombudsmans-review-complaint-handling-nhs-england-2011-12 (accessed: 7 March 2021).

Patients Association (2013) *Complaint Handling in NHS Trusts Signed Up to the CARE Campaign: Reality criteria and identification of best practice*. Harrow: The Patients Association.

Porter-O'Grady, T. (2004) Overview: Shared governance: Is it a model for nurses to gain control over their practice?, *Online Journal of Issues in Nursing*, 9 (1). Available at: https://ojin.nursingworld.org/MainMenuCategories/ANAMarketplace/ANAPeriodicals/OJIN/TableofContents/Volume92004/No1Jan04/Overview.html (accessed: 7 March 2021).

Salzburg Statement on Shared Decision-Making (2011) *British Medical Journal*, 342: d1745. Available at: https://doi.org/10.1136/bmj.d1745.

Som, C. (2004) Clinical governance: A fresh look at its definition, *Clinical Governance: An International Journal*, 9 (2): 87–90.

Stigglebout, A.M., Van der Weijden, T., De Wit, M.P.T., Frosch, D., Legare, F., Montori, V.M. *et al.* (2012) Shared decision-making: Really putting patients at the centre of healthcare, *British Medical Journal*, 344: e256. Available at: https://doi.org/10.1136/bmj.e256.

Sullivan, R., Barnby, E., and Graham, S. (2020) Evaluation of a modified version of the Norton Scale for use as a pressure injury risk assessment instrument in critical care, *Journal of Wound Ostomy and Continence Nursing*, 47 (3): 224–229.

Wei, M., Wu, L., Chen, Y., Fu, Q., Chen, W., and Yang, D. (2020) Predictive validity of the Braden scale for pressure ulcer risk in critical care: A meta-analysis, *Nursing in Critical Care*, 25 (3): 165–170.

Williams, S., Turner, A.M., and Beadle, H. (2018) Experience-based co-design to improve a pulmonary rehabilitation programme, *International Journal of Health Care Quality Assurance*, 32 (5): 778–787.

World Health Organization (WHO) (2006) *Quality of Care: A process for making strategic choices in health systems*. Geneva: WHO.

8 Evaluating quality care through audit

Mary Gottwald and Gail E. Lansdown

Chapter contents

- Learning objectives
- Introduction
- Clinical audit
- Audit versus research
- Audit versus quality improvement
- Central principles of clinical audit
- Designing audit
- The audit cycle
- Advantages, disadvantages, and barriers to clinical audit
- Approaches to audit
- Key points summary
- Implications for practice
- End-of-chapter questions
- References

Learning objectives

By the end of this chapter, the reader will be better able to:

- Identify the rationale for clinical audit
- Apply the audit cycle to practice
- Recognize barriers to clinical audit
- Recognize criteria for successful audit

Introduction

Chapter 1 highlighted a number of high-profile cases in the UK that led to public inquiries focusing on the failure of the NHS. The outcome of these inquiries led to a loss of trust in the NHS. Chapter 2 went on to discuss some examples where the quality of care could be called into question. Chapter 6 focused on the importance of evidence-based practice (EBP) and values-based practice (VBP), and this chapter will focus on how audit can be used to identify where there is a lack of quality care but also provide evidence for excellent care provision. However, it is important to recognize that EBP and audit have different functions. In 2013, one of the key recommendations from the Francis Report was that audit of practice should be mandatory. The Care Quality Commission (CQC) use audit as part of their performance measures and state that as part of the Health and Social Care Act (2008) (Regulated Activities) Regulations 2014: Regulation 17, organizations must demonstrate that they have effective auditing systems in place.

As the world has battled with the COVID-19 pandemic, audit has become even more important to ensure quality of care. The UK NHS and organizations globally are accountable for their decisions during the pandemic and have been forced to move away from the business-as-usual model to modified procedures. These modified procedures should be subject to the same oversight and scrutiny mechanisms. The use of technology has been key to enable effective decision-making, and to reduce the risk of claims or other legal challenges. All urgent decisions relating to COVID-19 should be appropriately documented to ensure a robust audit trail.

There has been a much greater use of technology during the pandemic, with remote consultations via mobile phone, messaging with a personal mobile phone using applications such as WhatsApp, video conferencing using a personal device, home working, email, and so on. The Information Commissioner's Office (ICO) and NHSX (teams from the Department of Health and Social Care, NHS England, and NHS Improvement) has produced guidance on information governance obligations and highlighted the importance of data-sharing within the health and social care sector. However, to ensure an appropriate audit trail, all patient contact entailing information technologies should be noted in the patient record.

Clinical audit

In the UK, the key aim of the Darzi Report (Department of Health, 2008) (see Chapter 1) was to improve the quality of care through the management of risk reduction. Results from clinical audits can identify these improvements as well as identify any reasons for lack of improvement. Audit can be used to benchmark organizations against similar organizations. This could result in extra demands and pressures being imposed on teams to improve, but might also be motivating for staff "if a gold standard is achieved" (Paskins *et al.*, 2010: 204).

Clinical audit is not a new concept and over time healthcare organizations have been scrutinized both internally and externally. In 1997, with the introduction of clinical governance, clinical audit became an integral part of professional practice. It is a quality improvement cycle, the key driver of which is to measure high-quality healthcare against agreed standards (Crabtree, Sundararaj, and Pease, 2020). Consequently, audit is now adopted by all health and social care professions that have a duty to conform to audit processes (Cowan, 2002; Sale, 2005; Clouston and Westcott, 2005; Benjamin, 2008; Boyle and Keep, 2018). Audit is a quality improvement process that was first introduced to the NHS by the 1989 White Paper, *Working for Patients* (Department of Health, 1989), and became mandatory for all hospital doctors in 1998 (Department of Health, 1998).

Audit is one methodology that can be used to evaluate quality improvement programmes. The Healthcare Quality Improvement Partnership (HQIP, 2020: 4) defines audit as:

> *A quality improvement cycle that involves measurement of the effectiveness of healthcare against agreed and proven standards for high quality and taking action to bring practice in line with these standards so as to improve the quality of care and health outcomes.*

HQIP (2020) remind us that audit should be a planned process and a continuous aspect of practice evaluation. Hospital board management therefore needs to have clear strategies in place to facilitate the implementation of this process. One of the key strategies is that organizations need to engage service users and the public in the evaluation of practice and enable their voices to be heard (Chapter 1). To this end, training in clinical audit may be required for service users and the public as well as staff. Results from audit need to be shared with stakeholders and action plans agreed to facilitate changes in practice. These changes need to be continuously scrutinized and evaluated to ensure sustained improvement in the quality of care provided.

Activity 8.1

Access *Best Practice in Clinical Audit* (HQIP, 2020) at the following link:

https://www.hqip.org.uk/wp-content/uploads/2020/05/FINAL-Best-Practice-in-Clinical-Audit-2020.pdf (accessed: 7 March 2021)

Although this link relates to the UK, HQIP identifies some important aspects around audit that must be considered in all healthcare practice.

- What strategies are used in your organization to ensure practice is evaluated through audit?
- Are you involved in audit and, if so, was further training provided by your organization?
- Which audit approaches are used within your organization, for example random audit, focused audit, retrospective audit, external audit, or internal audit?
- Are you informed about the results of audits that have taken place on your ward or in your organization?

We introduced the audit cycle in Chapter 3 and the above activity asks whether you have been involved with the audit process or whether you have been informed about the results of an audit that has taken place on your ward. Pederson *et al.* (2018) pose the question whether being given the results of an audit will increase motivation to continue to improve the quality of care provided. They carried out a naturalistic study in Norway using focus groups to collect qualitative data from staff working within mental health services, focusing on the audit and feedback cycle. In Chapter 4, we discussed evidence that highlights some staff will resist change and yet changing practice is key to the audit cycle.

Results from the Norwegian study showed that staff interviewed viewed audit along with feedback as a positive experience because it made them more cognisant of what was happening in practice (Pederson *et al.*, 2018). However, at times the everyday pressures of working within mental health services impinged on their ability to complete the audit and feedback cycle. Once staff are provided with feedback, the audit cycle must continue and it is essential that a new action plan is drawn up and that changes in practice are again evaluated. Participants in this study highlighted that action plans were not always followed through, therefore managers need to ensure that staff have followed the processes identified in the action plan. For example, one participant stated that if they were expected to read the national guidelines, managers needed to have a system in place that demonstrated members of staff had read them. We suggest that one useful way that this could occur would be through a CPD seminar, where staff are asked to share their concerns, viewpoints, and challenges when reading and adhering to national guidelines and share examples of how they are implementing guidelines in their practice.

For staff to be motivated to follow an action plan requires good leadership, such as transformational leadership (Lumbers, 2018), because leaders would then be able to demonstrate that they "own" the audit and feedback process, and staff would be assured that managers would facilitate them to implement the action plan. Staff interviewed in Pederson and colleagues' (2018) research felt that if they were more involved and supported with the audit and feedback process, they would be more motivated to adhere to any action plan.

Key points

- Completing the audit cycle is essential and must be a continuous process
- Staff need support and be given time to ensure they complete the audit cycle
- Providing feedback from audits can be motivating, especially when results show standards have been met

Audit versus research

Audit measures practice against standards and performance. Audit poses the question, "Are we doing the right thing in the right way?" Research, on the other hand, asks the question, "What is the right thing to do?" Table 8.1 highlights the differences between audit and research.

Table 8.1 The difference between audit and research

Research	Audit
Generates new knowledge	Current knowledge is used to best effect
Is initiated by researchers	Usually led by service providers
Is theory-driven (hypothesis-based)	Is practice-driven (standard-based)
Is often a one-off event	Is an ongoing process
Is large-scale for prolonged periods of time	Usually less largescale and prolonged than research
Often involves statistical analysis	Minimal statistical analysis
May involve randomly allocating service users to different treatment groups	Never involves randomly allocating service users to treatment groups
May involve administration of placebo	Never involves placebo
Often requires approval from an ethical committee	Never requires approval from an ethical committee

Adapted from: Dilnawaz, Mazhar, and Shaikh (2012).

Audit versus quality improvement

Audit and quality improvement are essentially the same, as they both examine healthcare standards and how to improve them. The difference lies in the fact that audits have a more formal standard to measure against and usually span a longer timeframe, for example they are undertaken every few months. Quality improvement, on the other hand, using a PDSA (Plan, Do, Study, Act) cycle (Christoff, 2018), can be undertaken weekly or even daily.

According to NICE, clinical audit "should be at the very heart of clinical governance systems" (2002: viii). Recently, there has been a move away from optional clinical audit activity to a more obligatory approach and hence clinical audit has become a pillar and formal part of the clinical governance framework in the UK and elsewhere. Chapter 5 presented the case for continued professional development (CPD) and because auditing clinical practice highlights areas of both good and poor practice, it enables professionals continuously to pursue best evidence-based practice (Chapter 6).

All the public inquiries discussed in Chapter 1 will have included an audit of the healthcare provided and will have made recommendations, some of which will have linked to audit. For example, the Bristol Royal Infirmary Inquiry (2001: 167) made 198 recommendations, three of which are specific to audit:

1 *Recommendation 143*: Audit should be central to organizational monitoring systems and processes

2 *Recommendation 144*: Audit must be supported by healthcare Trusts so that staff are provided with the necessary resources to carry out an audit

3 *Recommendation 145*: Clinical staff contracts stipulated the requirement to participate in audit

It is therefore imperative that staff understand what an audit involves. NICE (2002: 1) provide a clear definition of this:

> *Clinical audit is a quality improvement process that seeks to improve patient care and outcomes through systematic review of care against explicit criteria and the implementation of change. Aspects of the structure, processes, and outcomes of care are selected and systematically evaluated against explicit criteria. Where indicated changes are implemented at an individual, team or service level and further monitoring is used to confirm improvement in healthcare delivery.*

As this definition makes clear, audit is both a quality improvement and a change process based on the appraisal of current practice.

Donabedian (1966) suggested three aspects of performance:

1 Structure (what is needed)
2 Process (what is done)
3 Outcome of care (what is expected)

Audit usually falls into one of these, or may involve a combination of two or more. Examples of each of these are given in Table 8.2.

Audit involves examination of processes employed in healthcare to ensure that procedures are followed, standards are achieved, no impropriety occurs,

Table 8.2 Structure, process, and outcome audit

Structure	This relates to the resources that are considered essential so that organizations meet their strategic objectives, and will include aspects such as amenities, equipment, staffing, and skill mix
Process	This links to practice, clinical decision-making, assessment, prescribing, clinical interventions such as surgery, physiotherapy, and occupational therapy, and methods of record-keeping
Outcome	Outcome audit is linked to process audit and concerns the expected short- and long-term impact of healthcare provision. For example, the short-term impact of prescribing statins (process) to reduce cholesterol levels, will impact on the likelihood (outcome) of not having a heart attack or stroke in the long term

Adapted from: NICE (2002), Wright and Hill (2003), Benjamin (2008), and Donnellon *et al.* (2013).

stakeholders are optimally treated, and best value is obtained from the resources consumed (Sale, 2005). Audit involves measuring current practice against best practice and comparing what is being done against what should be done. Relevant changes required to improve the quality of care can be implemented and then re-audited to measure the final outcomes (Clouston and Westcott, 2005). Audit is not simply about identifying poor practice – it is also about identifying examples of good practice. It is important for teams to understand why practice is considered good, and conversely why some practices are considered not so good (Wright and Hill, 2003; Sale, 2005).

If the results of audit do identify poor practice, education and training at the team level (Chapter 5) becomes important, for example clinical guidelines and processes of care could be covered within workshops (Wright and Hill, 2003). Audit results can be influential in that they can lead an organization to review and change its practice (Paskins *et al.*, 2010). However, as identified in Chapter 4, changing practice is not always easy and therefore good leadership and teamwork are required.

It is important to be aware that clinical audit has a mixed reception amongst healthcare professionals and some government publications – *Good Doctors, Safer Patients* (Department of Health, 2006) and the *Assurance and Safety* White Paper (Department of Health, 2007) – concluded that clinical audit was falling short of its potential and thus needed to be strengthened.

NICE (2002) stipulates that for audit to be successful, the environment needs to be supportive and the methods used need to enable staff to engage in audit projects that enhance the provision of quality healthcare. If we return to the Department of Health's definition of clinical governance, we can see the importance of organizations creating supportive environments: "A framework through which organisations are accountable for continuously improving the quality of services and safeguarding high standards of care by creating an environment in which clinical care will flourish" (1998: 33).

Audit will not be successful if changes to practice are not implemented and the quality of services improved (Pickering and Thompson, 2003).

Central principles of clinical audit

Chapter 6 addressed evidence-based practice (EBP), and one tool that has been effective in supporting EBP is clinical audit. Audit sits in the fifth and final stage of the evidence cycle (Morrell and Harvey, 1999):

- Formulating a clinical question (using PICOT)
- Finding the evidence (searching the research literature)
- Critiquing the evidence (using a critiquing framework)
- Using the evidence to bring about change
- Evaluation using audit

Morrell and Harvey (1999) list the central principles of audit as:

- Professionally led
- An educational process
- A routine part of clinical practice
- Based on the setting of standards
- Generating results that can be used to improve the quality of care
- Involving management in both process and outcome
- Confidential at both the clinician and patient level
- Being informed by the views of both clinicians and patients

Furthermore, audit is central to clinical governance, which is illustrated in Figure 8.1. As can be seen, clinical audit is a quality improvement process that aims to improve patient care by systematically reviewing care against explicit criteria, leading to the implementation of change if necessary.

Figure 8.1 Linking audit to clinical governance

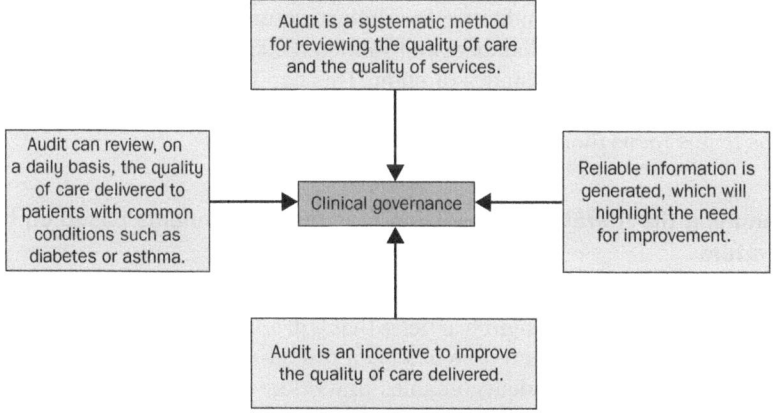

Designing audit

Chambers and Wakley (2005) suggest that the audit cycle has nine steps, three of which will be considered here. The remaining steps will be considered under the audit cycle.

Working with others, prioritizing, and selecting the audit topic

In order to engage healthcare professionals in audit, there need to be perceived benefits. The benefits may be to patients, colleagues, the organization, or the NHS. An audit topic is therefore likely to focus on an area that is

- High risk or
- High volume or
- High cost or
- Causes concern

If the audit focuses on a process or system, the benefits would need to have a bearing on efficiency or effectiveness. The outcome of all audits must have the potential to support improvements.

Chambers and Wakley (2005) suggest that the normal audit categories are:

- The frequency or volume of a service
- Risks associated with the provision of care
- Problems associated with the provision of care
- The effectiveness of the delivery of care
- The cost of delivering care

It is also important to remember that audit usually involves change and that communication is key.

As discussed earlier, audit may focus on structure, process, or outcome – or a combination thereof. Chambers and Wakley (2005) suggest an audit protocol that encapsulates all the stages of audit. This can be found on pages 18–21 of their ebook, *Clinical Audit in Primary Care*. This is a very useful tool that helps teams focus their ideas in preparing for an audit.

Examining the literature and setting reasonable standards based on the literature

Having defined a quality issue, it is important to interrogate the literature in a systematic way to find research articles that will address the issue. Readers are referred to Chapter 6 where this has been discussed in depth. Having a clear understanding of the evidence enables practitioners to set standards against which to monitor their practice.

Designing the audit: audit tools

The nursing profession was the first to implement standard-setting in the 1980s and therefore led the field in a systematic approach to monitoring quality against standards. Sale (2005: 199) describes a number of off-the-shelf, tried-and-tested nursing audit tools as she calls them. Three of the most commonly used are Qualpacs (Wandelt and Ager, 1974), Phaneuf's Nursing Audit (Phaneuf, 1976), and Monitor (Goldstone, Balt, and Callier, 1983).

Qualpacs

The Quality Patient Care Scale (Qualpacs) is an American tool and measures the quality of care received by the patient from the ward or unit nursing staff.

Consisting of 68 items, it measures the direct and indirect interaction of nursing staff with patients and is divided into six categories:

- Psychosocial (individual)   15 items
- Psychosocial (group)   8 items
- Physical   15 items
- General   15 items
- Communication   8 items
- Professional implications   7 items

Each item supplies prompts to assist in completing the audit. For example, under Psychosocial (individual), the first item is "Patient receives nurse's full attention". The prompts are as follows:

- The patient is appropriately responded to verbally and non-verbally, without being asked to repeat phrases
- Staff assume positions that will aid in observation and communication with patient
- Conversation of staff is restricted to the patient who is receiving care
- And so on

The prompts may be amended to suit the situation, as it is the item that is scored and not the prompt. Table 8.3 lists the advantages and disadvantages of Qualpac.

Phaneuf's Nursing Audit

This is a retrospective audit of the patient's records based on the assumption that good notes reflect good care. Using the seven functions of nursing

Table 8.3 Advantages and disadvantages of Qualpac

Advantages	Disadvantages
Rigorously tested and therefore reliable and valid	The values are American
Has been used in the UK, in the Nursing Development Unit in Oxford	Highly skilled and trained observers required
Data are provided by direct observation	Is time-consuming, both to administer and score
Uses more than one method of concurrent review	Observer bias can occur if observer is influenced by their own attitudes and expectations
By evaluating performance, provides nurses with an insight into their practice, thus improving patient care	May be subjective, it as relies on the professional judgement of the observer
Provides positive feedback to individuals and the team	

Adapted from: Sale (2005).

developed by Lesnik and Anderson (1955), Phaneuf designed 50 components to enable auditors to evaluate the quality of care from the medical records.

An audit committee with a minimum of five members will audit no more than 10 patients per month, with each audit taking approximately 15 minutes. Auditors will require training. As with Qualpac, this audit tool also has its advantages and disadvantages, which are shown in Table 8.4.

Monitor

Based on the Rush Medicus methodology (developed in Chicago between 1972 and 1975), Monitor was designed by North-West Region and Newcastle-upon-Tyne Polytechnic. A conceptual framework was developed to measure the nursing process, and patient needs and criteria were developed to evaluate quality of care within this framework. Six objectives representing the nursing process were identified:

1 A nursing plan is formulated
2 The physical needs of the patient are met
3 The physical, emotional, and social needs of the patient are met
4 Achievement of nursing care objectives is evaluated
5 Unit procedures are followed for the protection of all patients
6 The delivery of nursing care is facilitated by administrative and managerial services

Table 8.4 Advantages and disadvantages of Phaneuf's Nursing Audit

Advantages	Disadvantages
It can be used in all areas of nursing	Having been devised in the USA, it does not take account of British nursing, policies, politics, or procedures
The seven functions are easily understood	It cannot be used in areas where the nursing process has not been implemented
Scoring is reasonably simple	
The results are easy to understand	It is time-consuming
It assesses all those involved in recording care	Auditors need to be trained
It is useful if accurate records of care are kept	It only evaluates record-keeping and therefore helps to improve documentation rather than the delivery of care
	Based on assumptions – good records denote good care and what is done is documented and what is documented is done

Adapted from: Sale (2005).

Table 8.5 Advantages and disadvantages of Monitor

Advantages	Disadvantages
Information is collected from many areas, including documentation systems, management systems, the environment, delivery of care, and outcomes It gives feedback on quality of care It improves the performance of staff It gives an indication of patient satisfaction It can compare performance across wards and Trusts It measures the effectiveness of the nursing process It provides information that can be used in the future planning of training and development	Trained observers are required and this has a resource implication It requires the purchase of several copies of the document As the criteria are pre-set, there is no ownership of the process by the staff who are being measured There is no clear statement on its philosophy of nursing There are problems with observer reliability and subjectivity; this could be reduced with extensive training

Adapted from: Sale (2005).

Each of the six objectives contains a number of sub-objectives, and criteria were developed so that "yes", "no", or "not applicable" answers may be given. As with the two other audit tools discussed above, this one also has its advantages and disadvantages (Table 8.5).

The above are just three of a number of off-the-shelf tools to audit the nursing process. Although they each have their advantages and their disadvantages, one of their main advantages is that it can take a lot of time and effort to develop a good audit tool. However, the focus of these three tools is somewhat non-specific as they cover a wide range of criteria.

Not all audits require a validated tool as discussed above, and teams may choose to design the audit process themselves. This being the case, Chambers and Wakley's (2005) suggested audit protocol may be helpful.

Examining audit through a more up-to-date lens, Colquhoun *et al.* (2017) posit that audit and feedback (A&F) strategies have stagnated recently, as they have not been informed by behavioural and social science viewpoints. Undertaking semi-structured interviews with participants from a broad spectrum of disciplines (e.g. cognition, health and organizational psychology, medical decision-making and economics), and guided by descriptions of audit and feedback from the literature on healthcare, interviewees were questioned on how they might improve the A&F cycle.

Colquhoun *et al.* (2017) conducted 28 interviews and identified 313 hypotheses, which were placed into 30 themes. Overall, they demonstrated that the development and evaluation of A&F is driven by the intuition of individual investigators. They suggest a more theory-guided approach, which requires more research to further guide the evolution of A&F.

The audit cycle

Having chosen a relevant tool or designed an audit tool, the next stage is to carry out the audit. In order for quality improvement programmes to be successful, the process of audit needs to be continuous and cyclical, as illustrated in Figure 8.2. At the local level, once standards have been met, teams need to re-audit, set higher standards, and improve the level of quality further. At a wider level, the audit process may involve healthcare services within a specific region or even nationally.

Each stage of the audit cycle illustrated in Figure 8.2 will now be discussed in more depth.

Figure 8.2 The audit cycle

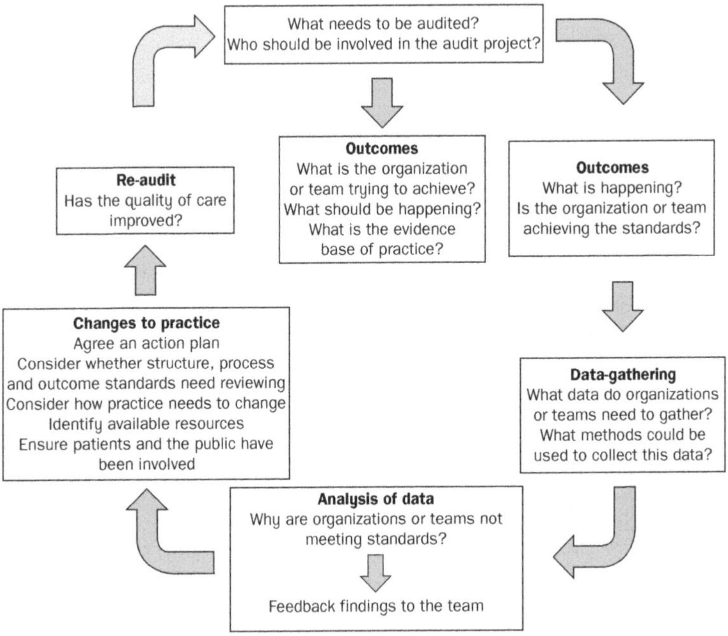

Adapted from: NICE (2002), Wright and Hill (2003), Benjamin (2008).

Stage 1: What needs to be audited and who needs to be involved?

Clinical audit is the method used to evaluate performance against evidence-based standards. Therefore, the aspect of audit that needs to be considered should be a quality issue where there is good evidence available on what comprises good quality care. For example, evidence available in relation to treatment and prevention of pressure ulcers, hospital-acquired infections, or medication errors (see Activity 8.2 below). If this evidence is limited, teams will find it difficult to identify standards that ensure best practice

(Wright and Hill, 2003; McSherry and Pearce, 2011). The clinical aspect chosen for audit should also link to national standards such as those identified by the National Institute for Health and Care Excellence up to January 2021 (NICE, 2021).

Each organization will have a clinical audit lead who will need to work alongside everybody who is involved in patient care, including health and social care professionals, stakeholders, service users, and patients. Everyone involved with either delivering or experiencing healthcare needs to be included in discussions related to which aspects of clinical practice ought to be audited. As well as involving relevant individuals in discussions, auditors can gather data through records of complaints (Chapter 7), risk management data (Chapter 7), significant events (near misses), patient satisfaction surveys, interviews (NICE, 2002; Pickering and Thompson, 2003), or via the Patient Voices Programme (Chapter 1).

If there have been a number of complaints, for example in relation to long waiting times in the A&E department, the teams may choose to carry out an audit so that causes can be identified. This could also involve setting up a quality circle, where stakeholders, patients, and service users can be involved. Together they might discuss what to include in the audit, how the audit will be carried out, and what responsibilities each should take. During a quality circle meeting, teams could also use fishbone analysis to identify the causes of poor quality care (Chapter 3). The Healthcare Quality Improvement Partnership (HQIP, 2020) states that stakeholders must be included in the audit process. Organizations may choose to also include stakeholders in their discussions on which quality issues to audit, thereby involving them in the first stage of the audit process.

As well as choosing topics that link to the evidence base of practice, topics need to link to the strategic objectives and organizational priorities (Benjamin, 2008). Organizations and teams may carry out significant events analysis, which could lead to the decision for a clinical audit being implemented. They will have to prioritize and it may be that the clinical governance committee or quality improvement committee makes the final decisions on which aspects of clinical practice will undergo clinical audit (NICE, 2002).

Activity 8.2

Explore the following links (all accessed: 7 March 2021):

http://www.thecochranelibrary.com/view/0/index.html
http://www.nice.org.uk
http://www.evidence.nhs.uk

These links will identify literature and evidence-based guidelines, for example NICE Clinical Guideline CG179: Pressure Ulcers (NICE, 2014). This guideline provides guidance on risk assessment, prevention, and treatment of pressure ulcers for all age groups. Practice can be compared with standard statements in the guidelines.

Activity 8.3

We have emphasized above the importance of engaging service users with the audit process and the importance for them to be able to share their experiences. Explore the following links, where you can access videos illustrating real-life patient experiences:

http://healthtalkonline.org (accessed: 7 March 2021)
http://healthtalkonline.org/young-peoples-experiences (accessed: 7 March 2021)

The following links are specific examples of patients sharing their experiences (all accessed: 7 March 2021):

- Asperger's syndrome
  https://healthtalk.org/life-autism-spectrum/overview
- Depression
  https://healthtalk.org/depression/overview
- Mental health: ethnic minority carers' experiences
  https://healthtalk.org/mental-health-ethnic-minority-carers-experiences/overview
- Rheumatoid arthritis
  https://healthtalk.org/rheumatoid-arthritis/overview
- Intensive care
  https://healthtalk.org/intensive-care-patients-experiences/overview

Stage 2: Outcomes

In order to meet the outcomes, organizations and teams need to have identified measurable standards. These audit criteria are explicit statements that define an outcome that can be measured. They should relate to important aspects of care and be derived from the best available evidence. Having explicit selection criteria will ensure that the data collected is precise and that only essential information is gathered.

Standards should relate to important standards that are thresholds of the expected compliance for each criterion and they should be based on the best evidence available. A minimum standard describes the lowest acceptable standard of performance and is often used as the cut-off for acceptable and unacceptable performance. "Ideal standards describe the care it should be possible to give under ideal conditions, with no constraints" (Anderson, cited in Benjamin, 2008: 1244). Unfortunately, such standards cannot usually be achieved. Whilst most people would like to see ideal standards – and many audit teams write such standards – in the real world of healthcare in the twenty-first century, they may be unrealistic. The development of standards will usually involve a combination of clinical experience and a review of the available evidence.

To understand whether these standards are being achieved within realistic timeframes, there is a requisite that standards be monitored. Sale (2005: 54) proposes that there is a difference between the monitoring of standards and auditing standards. Monitoring standards identifies any gaps and provides teams with a "snapshot" of whether quality care is being provided because the standards have been met. A "detailed portrait" and clinical audit are required when there are unmet aspects of the standards.

Activity 8.4

NICE identifies quality standards for quality improvement in health and social care. Whilst not mandatory they are useful when planning services to ensure the best possible care.

https://www.nice.org.uk/standards-and-indicators (accessed: 7 March 2021)

The CQC also provide information on the fundamental standards that should be achieved:

https://www.cqc.org.uk/what-we-do/how-we-do-our-job/fundamental-standards (accessed: 7 March 2021)

Reflect on your practice. Choose two standards from above and list three ways in which you could ensure that your practice meets these standards.

Stage 3: Data-gathering

Data is in the main gathered through the examination of patient case records, and therefore ethical principles such as anonymity and confidentiality must be respected (Swage, 2004). Wright and Hill (2003: 103) make three suggestions that help this process:

1 *Define and agree what information is required*: In relation to auditing the quality of care, data on "diagnosis, co-morbidity, interventions, and complications" would be valuable

2 *Design and pilot an audit proforma*: It is important to carry out a pilot to ensure the data is relevant and easy to analyse (Hicks, 2004)

3 *Select the sample*: Avoiding bias within audit is crucial and therefore sampling methods should either (a) include all patient records within a given time period, or (b) include a random sample, for example using random number tables (Hicks, 2004). The sample selected should be one that reflects the characteristics of the population from which it has been drawn. Data collected may be retrospective, concurrent, or prospective. The differences between these are highlighted in Table 8.6.

Table 8.6 Data collection

Categories	Retrospective	Prospective	Concurrent
Definition	Data collected by looking back over practice, i.e. patients that have been discharged	Data collected from this point onwards, starting at a future date. In the future, either a retrospective or concurrent audit will be carried out	Data are collected on patients who are still in hospital or receiving care, thus the audit is concurrent with actual patient care
When to use	When looking at what has happened in a chosen topic area	Data currently not available; data of poor quality	When patients care plans need to be reviewed
Advantages	Can be faster; provides a baseline	Avoids using poor data; allows design of clear data collection	The patient benefits at the time of the audit because problems are identified at the time of care
Disadvantages	Past service users do not benefit	No baseline provided; can be time-consuming	Time-consuming and costly to implement

Adapted from: Hicks (2004), Dilnawaz *et al.* (2012).

Activity 8.5

If you are going to lead an audit project, the following questions ought to be considered:

- Who is going to collect the data?
- How is the data going to be collected?
- Who will develop the data collection proforma?
- Who will pilot the proforma and amend it if needed?
- What challenges do you envisage?
- What support would you need to overcome these challenges?

Stage 4: Analysis of data

Once data have been collected, they need to be compared with the standards and criteria set and the evidence base of practice as identified by agreed national standards, such as the NICE (2021) and CQC standards and indicators mentioned above. Following the analysis, the findings must be disseminated to the team. Pederson *et al.* (2018) highlight that when findings were disseminated, teams were more motivated to engage with the audit cycle and continually develop and improve their practice.

Standards could include a reduction in errors such as medication errors, hospital-acquired infections, or pressure ulcers, and standard statements may be written as follows:

> *By the end of 2022, there will be a 40% reduction in medication errors.*

The analysis of data can result in both positive and negative outcomes – for example, if a 60% reduction in medication errors has been achieved, this demonstrates a clear improvement in patient care. On the other hand, if a 35% reduction is identified, this conveys a need to continue to focus on improving processes such as the prescription of medication. When setting standards, it is important to consider the percentage, because setting too high a standard (100%) may not be realistic or achievable, so setting an optimum standard is better. Once a standard of, say, 40% has been achieved, a higher percentage can be agreed and once that percentage is achieved, the standard can be set even higher. This ensures continuous quality improvement.

Stage 5: Changing practice to improve the quality of care

This can be the most challenging part of the audit cycle because the results of the data analysis are likely to require a change in practice and, as discussed in Chapter 4, this can be a difficult experience for practitioners. Once areas of poor practice have been identified, discussions can take place on how to manage the poor performance of a team or individual (Donnellon, Hurford, and Cox, 2013). Donnellon *et al.* (2013) and Pederson *et al.* (2018) suggest that if formative feedback is provided to individuals or teams, that will encourage reflection on practice, and if support is given that facilitates the development of their knowledge, skills, and clinical decision-making, practice and engagement with the audit cycle will be enhanced. CPD programmes (Chapter 5) are an important aspect of changing practice. Agreeing an action plan will facilitate changes to practice and will enable teams to monitor progress in relation to agreed objectives, strategies, and actions. The action plan needs to include SMART objectives, what the tasks are, and who is responsible for each of those tasks.

Stage 6: Re-audit

The last stage of the audit cycle involves repeating the audit. This audit must be carried out in the same way as the initial audit to ensure that accurate and valid comparisons can be made. The results from the re-audit will identify whether changes have been made, standards have been met and maintained, and the quality of healthcare provision improved. Re-auditing can also demonstrate whether there is an increasing trend in meeting required standards (Swage, 2004; Donnellon *et al.*, 2013; HQIP, 2020). It is important that teams agree further changes and agree to another audit at a later date. Having said this, it is important to be mindful that perhaps too many audits are conducted (Boyle and Keep, 2018) and therefore whilst there is a need to engage staff, audits should be more focused, allowing more time for specific evaluations of interventions to be carried out. This would lead to more successful quality improvement programmes.

Advantages, disadvantages, and barriers to clinical audit

Advantages and disadvantages

In order to review the benefits and disadvantages of clinical audit, Johnston *et al.* (2000) carried out a systematic review of articles retrieved from the Medline and CINAHL databases for the years 1992 to 1997. In total, 93 articles were reviewed, across a range of audit processes, including individual audit projects and retrospective reviews of departmental audit programmes at the interface between primary and secondary care. The experiences of all staff grades, from medical consultants to professionals allied to medicine and from staff involved in both unidisciplinary and multidisciplinary care, were collected. A summary of the findings is given in Table 8.7.

Garg, Singhal, and Neelam also identify some benefits for the auditor. Carrying out an audit provides staff with a chance to develop their "skills in project management, team-working, reflective practice, clinical governance and service development" (2010: 49).

Table 8.7 Advantages and disadvantages of clinical audit

Advantages	Disadvantages
Improved communication across clinical groups	Reduced clinical ownership
	Fear of litigation
Improved patient care	Professional isolation
Increased professional satisfaction	Suspicions due to hierarchy and
Improved administration	territorialism

Barriers

Having discussed the pros and cons of a clinical audit, let us look at a number of barriers to implementing it in the workplace. Chambers and Wakley (2005) provide the following barriers to audit:

- Negative attitudes and an unwillingness to participate
- A lack of willingness on the part of the team as a whole to get involved (a multidisciplinary approach is required)
- Audit is seen as an extra undertaking
- Overwhelmed healthcare practitioners feel they have insufficient time
- Lack of resources, especially time
- Lack of training in audit and evidence-based skills
- Patients and service users unwilling to take part
- Lack of communication
- Imbalance between an individual's desire to audit and the needs of the service
- Failure to provide a supportive climate for audit, and sensitivity as some individuals may feel uncomfortable that their performance is being monitored
- Fear of and resistance to change
- Failure to complete the audit cycle
- The cost of carrying out audit and implementing change

Activity 8.6

Think of the last time you were involved in an audit. Did any of the barriers listed above impede the process?

Johnston *et al.* (2000: 23) surmised that there are five main barriers to clinical audit:

1 Lack of resources
2 Lack of expertise/advice in design and analysis
3 Difficulties between groups and group members
4 Lack of an overall plan for audit
5 Organizational hindrance

In contrast, Johnston *et al.* (2000) found the key factors supporting audit to be:

- Modern medical records systems
- Effective training
- Motivated and dedicated staff
- Good leadership
- Protected time
- Dialogue between purchasers and providers
- Mechanisms to support data collection, including IT systems

- Strategy and planning
- High levels of audit activity, with monitoring and reporting integral to the process
- Protective time for clinicians
- A supportive organization

Activity 8.7

Bearing in mind that Johnston and colleagues' article was published in 2000, which, if any, of the disadvantages and barriers still exist in your place of work?

The recommendation of Johnston *et al.* (2000) to seek the opinions of clinicians on the process of a new audit was picked up by Paskins *et al.* in 2010. Examining an annual regional rheumatology audit that has been running in the West Midlands since 2000, they found that this was considered an efficient use of resources and had unexpected educational benefits whilst promoting good relationships across the region.

Garg *et al.* (2010) focused their research on why staff do not become engaged in the audit process. They identified some of the difficulties and barriers trainee doctors experienced when carrying out clinical audit, and these are illustrated in Table 8.8. This nationwide UK study involved an online survey of student doctors working within psychiatry. In total, 504 doctors responded to the questionnaire, a response rate of 89%; this response rate is high and therefore results can be deemed to be relevant (Denscombe, 2010). Altogether, the respondents had been involved in 2,267 audits. However, the completion rate of the audit cycle, in particular completion of stage 6 as discussed above, was considered low.

Boyle and Keep (2018) highlight the importance of audit standards measuring the processes that are in place in an organization, the structure of the organization, and the outcomes of the organization. These are three of the key attributes of clinical governance proposed by Som (2004) and addressed in Chapter 1. Boyle and Keep (2018) refer to the barriers identified by Johnston *et al.* (2000) and discussed above. They also question whether audits, as a quality assurance process, lead to better patient safety and improved outcomes. They posit that carrying out numerous audits takes time, time that could instead be devoted to improving the quality of patient care. They conclude that there is a need to engage staff, carry out more focused audits, and that specific evaluation of interventions would lead to more successful quality improvement programmes.

In a study that met the WHO and World Bank's (2017) Sustainable Development Goals (SDG 3 – good health and wellbeing, as previously discussed in the rationale for this book), Rousseva *et al.* (2020) undertook a qualitative evidence synthesis of healthcare workers' views on audit to improve the quality of maternal and newborn healthcare in low- and middle-income countries. Having searched the PubMed, CINAHL, and Global Health databases, 19 papers were identified and included in their review, most from sub-Saharan Africa. Healthcare workers who took part in the study mostly held positive views of audit and were committed to the process. The majority of them had a positive experience of being part of the audit process. The main barriers to taking part in clinical audit were seen to be the presence of a blame culture, as opposed to a just culture, insufficient training and time, and a lack of resources. The barriers outlined in this systematic review are very similar to those found in the UK and elsewhere.

Table 8.8 Barriers to getting involved in clinical audit

Time	Work-based pressures on top of routine clinical activities impacted on available time to carry out an audit. Examples cited included time taken to attend CPD courses, time to study for exams, and time to complete job applications and attend for interviews. Time was not specifically allocated for the audit and so had to be carried out within rostered clinical hours and often trainee doctors were not in placement long enough to complete the audit cycle
Lack of support	Lack of training to carry out an audit Lack of support from medical records departments in providing information Management, senior clinicians, and clinical governance team members absent at audit meetings
Lack of motivation	Respondents identified that if team members disagreed with the audit findings, were resistant to changing practice following the outcome of the audit, or if recommendations were not implemented, then the auditors lost motivation to carry out further audits
Poor communication	Poor communication leading to conflict within teams prevented changes to practice being carried forward. Results of audits were not always clearly disseminated and therefore teams were not aware of the impact of changing practice on improved quality of patient care

Adapted from: Garg *et al*. (2010).

Activity 8.8

Compare the findings of Chalmers and Wakley (2005) to those of Garg *et al*. (2010). Bearing in mind that these authors were writing five years apart, what reduction in barriers, if any, can you see?

Approaches to audit

Having discussed what needs to be considered when designing an audit tool, the audit cycle, barriers to audit, and the strengths and limitations of audit, Table 8.9 illustrates a number of approaches to audit that teams and individuals ought to consider.

Table 8.9 Approaches to audit

Self-audit	Using the evidence (as discussed in Chapter 6) to ensure practice is up to date and evidence-based
Peer audit	Asking a colleague to observe practice to ensure that it meets set standards
Critical incident audit	The multidisciplinary team discusses anonymous cases that have either caused concern or had an unexpected outcome
Supervisory audit	Often undertaken as part of the appraisal or professional development review, in which the line manager audits achievements against set standards
Internal audit	Provides independent assurance that an organization's risk management, governance, and internal control processes are operating effectively. Auditors report to the board and senior management
External audit	Gives opinion on the credibility and reliability of financial reports to the organization's stakeholders. Additionally, external bodies such as the Care Quality Commission (CQC) will audit to ensure that quality standards are met
Continuous audit	Standards are audited continuously
Random audit	Standards are randomly selected and audited
Focused audit	A specific area for audit is chosen
Retrospective audit	Involves audit of medical records once a patient has been discharged
Non-criterion-based audit	A broader audit that goes beyond meeting agreed standards

Adapted from: Sale (2005).

Activity 8.9

Thinking about when you have been involved in audit, which of the approaches in Table 8.9 have been utilized by your organization?

Resources

The Healthcare Quality Improvement Partnership (HQIP) was established in April 2008 to promote quality in healthcare and thereby increase the impact that clinical audit has on healthcare quality in England and Wales. Guidance, training, and support for clinical audit can be accessed at:

http://www.hqip.org.uk/guidance-support (accessed: 7 March 2021)

Key points summary

Audit is both a quality improvement and a change process based on the appraisal of current practice. It identifies both excellent practice as well as the need to improve practice. Audit sits in the fifth and final stage of the evidence cycle and all health and social care professionals have a duty to conform to the audit process. Although there are a number of off-the-shelf audit tools, many teams decide to design their own. If that is the case, Chambers and Wakley's (2005) protocol may be useful and can be used in conjunction with the audit cycle shown in Figure 8.2. Teams need also to consider the advantages, disadvantages, and barriers to implementing an audit.

Implications for practice

- Audit should be embraced and seen as a part of everyday practice
- It is essential that you choose the right audit tool to evaluate the quality issue
- An appropriate audit approach must be selected (Table 8.9)
- There are advantages and disadvantages to audit

End-of-chapter questions

1 What approach would you use when there has been an unexpected outcome to treatment given?
2 When might you undertake a retrospective audit?
3 What are the advantages of audit?
4 Name three barriers to clinical audit.

See the Appendix on page 256 for suggested answers to these questions.

References

Benjamin, A. (2008) Audit: How to do it in practice, *British Medical Journal*, 336 (7655): 1241–1245. Available at: https://doi.org/10.1136/bmj.39527.628322.AD.

Boyle, A. and Keep, J. (2018) Clinical audit does not work, is quality improvement any better?, *British Journal of Hospital Medicine*, 79(9): 508–510.

Bristol Royal Infirmary Inquiry (2001) *The Report of the Public Inquiry into Children's Heart Surgery at the Bristol Royal Infirmary 1984–1995: Learning from Bristol.* Bristol: Bristol Royal Infirmary Inquiry.

Chambers, R. and Wakley, G. (2005) *Clinical Audit in Primary Care: Demonstrating quality and outcomes.* Oxford: Radcliffe.

Christoff, P. (2018) Running PDSA cycles, *Current Problems in Pediatric and Adolescent Health Care*, 48 (8): 198–201.

Clouston, T. and Westcott, L. (2005) *Working in Health and Social Care: An introduction for allied health professionals.* London: Elsevier Churchill Livingstone.

Colquhoun, H.L., Carroll, K., Eva, K.W., Grimshaw, J.M., Ivers, N., Michie, S. *et al.* (2017) Advancing the literature on designing audit and feedback interventions: Identifying theory-informed hypotheses, *Implementation Science*, 12: 117. Available at: https://doi.org/10.1186/s13012-017-0646-0.

Cowan, P. (2002) Clinical risk management: The role of clinical audit in risk reduction, *British Journal of Clinical Governance*, 7 (3): 220–223.

Crabtree, A., Sundararaj, J.J., and Pease, N. (2020) Clinical audit? – invaluable!, *British Medical Journal Supportive and Palliative Care*, 10 (2): 213–215.

Denscombe, M. (2010) *The Good Research Guide: For small-scale social research projects.* Maidenhead: Open University Press.

Department of Health (1989) *Working for Patients*, Cm 555. London: HMSO.

Department of Health (1998) *A First Class Service: Quality in the new NHS.* Available at: http://webarchive.nationalarchives.gov.uk/+/www.dh.gov.uk/en/publicationsandstatistics/publications/publicationspolicyand-guidance/dh_4006902 (accessed: 7 March 2021).

Department of Health (2006) *Good Doctors, Safer Patients: Proposals to strengthen the system to assure and improve the performance of doctors and to protect the safety of patients.* London: HMSO.

Department of Health (2007) *Trust, Assurance and Safety: The regulation of health professionals.* London: HMSO.

Department of Health (2008) *High Quality Care for All: NHS next stage review final report.* Available at: http://www.official-documents.gov.uk/document/cm74/7432/7432.pdf (accessed: 7 March 2021).

Dilnawaz, M., Mazhar, H., and Shaikh, Z.I. (2012) Clinical audit: A simplified approach, *Journal of Pakistan Association of Dermatologists*, 22 (4): 358–362.

Donabedian, A. (1966) Evaluating the quality of care, *Milbank Quarterly*, 44: 166–204.

Donnellon, K., Hurford, G., and Cox, D. (2013) It's good to talk: Auditing clinicians' interactions with patients in a primary care setting, *Clinical Governance: An International Journal*, 18 (3): 220–227.

Francis Report (2013) *Report of the Mid Staffordshire NHS Trust Foundation Trust Public Inquiry.* London: HMSO.

Garg, D., Singhal, A., and Neelam, K. (2010) Clinical audits by trainee doctors: Obstacles and solutions, *Clinical Governance: An International Journal*, 17 (1): 45–53.

Goldstone, L.A., Balt, J.A., and Callier, M. (1983) *Monitor: An index of the quality of nursing care for acute medical and surgical wards.* Newcastle-upon-Tyne: Polytechnic Products.

Health and Social Care Act (2008) Available at: https://services.parliament.uk/bills/2007-08/healthandsocialcare.html (accessed: 7 March 2021).

Healthcare Quality Improvement Partnership (HQIP) (2020) *Best Practice in Clinical Audit*. London: HQIP.

Hicks, C. (2004) *Research Methods for Clinical Therapists: Applied project design and analysis*. London: Churchill Livingstone.

Johnston, G., Crombie, J.K., Davies, H.T.O., Alder, E.M., and Millard, A. (2000) Reviewing audit: Barriers and facilitating factors for effective clinical audit, *Quality in Health-care*, 9 (1): 23–36.

Lesnik, M.J. and Anderson, B.E. (1955) *Nursing Practice and the Law*, 2nd edition. Philadelphia, PA: Lippincott.

Lumbers, M. (2018) Approaches to leadership and managing change in the NHS, *British Journal of Nursing*, 27 (10): 554–558.

McSherry, R. and Pearce, P. (2011) *Clinical Governance: A guide to implementation for healthcare professionals*. Oxford: Blackwell.

Morrell, C. and Harvey, G. (1999) *The Clinical Audit Handbook: Improving the quality of healthcare*. Oxford: Baillière Tindall.

NICE (2002) *Principles of Best Practice in Clinical Audit*. Oxford: Radcliffe Medical Press.

NICE (2014) *Pressure Ulcers: Prevention and management*, Clinical Guideline CG179. Available at: https://www.nice.org.uk/guidance/cg179 (accessed: 25 June 2021).

NICE (2021) *Audit and Service Improvement*. Available at: https://www.nice.org.uk/about/what-we-do/into-practice/audit-and-service-improvement (accessed: 7 March 2021).

Paskins, Z., John, H., Hassel, A., and Rowe, I. (2010) The perceived advantages and disadvantages of regional audit: A qualitative study, *Clinical Governance: An International Journal*, 15 (3): 200–209.

Pederson, M., Landheim, A., Moller, M., and Lien, L. (2018) Audit and feedback in mental healthcare: Staff experiences, *Journal of Health Care Quality Assurance*, 31 (7): 822–833.

Phaneuf, M.C. (1976) *The Nursing Audit: Self-regulation in nursing practice*. New York: Appleton-Century-Crofts.

Pickering, S. and Thompson, J. (2003) *Clinical Governance and Best Value*. London: Churchill Livingstone.

Rousseva, C., Lammath, V., Tancred, T., and Smith, H. (2020) Health workers' views on audit in maternal and newborn healthcare in LMICs: A qualitative evidence synthesis, *Tropical Medicine and International Health*, 5 (5): 525–539.

Sale, D. (2005) *Understanding Clinical Governance and Quality Assurance: Making it happen*. Basingstoke: Palgrave Macmillan.

Som, C. (2004) Clinical governance: A fresh look at its definition, *Clinical Governance: An International Journal*, 9 (2): 87–90.

Swage, T. (2004) *Clinical Governance in Healthcare Practice*. London: Butterworth Heinemann.

Wandelt, M.A. and Ager, J.W. (1974) *Quality Patient Care Scale*. New York: Appleton-Century-Crofts.

World Health Organization and The World Bank (2017) *Tracking Universal Health Coverage: 2017 global monitoring report*. Available at: http://documents1.world-bank.org/curated/en/640121513095868125/pdf/122029-WP-REVISED-PUBLIC.pdf (accessed: 7 March 2021).

Wright, J. and Hill, P. (2003) *Clinical Governance*. London: Churchill Livingstone.

Conclusion

We hope that this book has provided you with further insight regarding the importance of clinical governance and how clinical governance should underpin the practice of everyone working in a healthcare setting – anywhere in the world, regardless of their role. All of us, whether working in a clinical or non-clinical capacity, are responsible for the continuous improvement of practice and the implementation of the clinical governance agenda.

In the UK, the quality of healthcare is still very much an issue, despite regular government involvement since the 1990s, the genesis of clinical governance, and the requirement to appoint clinical governance leads. This was evident in the recent failings at Shrewsbury and Telford NHS Trust, which were highlighted in The Ockenden Report (2020). The World Health Organization has urged healthcare providers to be mindful of clinical governance. The World Bank and WHO have made universal health coverage a priority, and state in particular that services provided need to be of sufficient quality to lead to improvements in health throughout the world.

The inquiries that we have discussed in this book acknowledge that workloads are heavy, resources are limited, and staffing levels are not always optimal. However, this should not allow us to become complacent. We accept that the creation of clinical governance leads was an important first step in raising awareness of how the clinical governance agenda could improve the quality of healthcare provision. But what was good enough in the early days of clinical governance is no longer good enough.

We believe that in order for organizations to become learning organizations, the application of two clinical governance strategies must be at the heart of everyone's practice regardless of their role. These strategies are, first, education and training at the individual, team, and organizational levels, and secondly, evidence- and values-based practice (EBP and VBP).

At the most basic level, organizations have a duty to provide education and training so that individuals have an understanding of how to search for and critique literature relevant to their practice. This can be supported further at the team level through journal clubs and critical incident (including complaints) discussions. At the organizational level, healthcare providers have a responsibility to ensure employees have an understanding of the clinical governance agenda and provide relevant CPD opportunities for all staff, regardless of level.

All clinical staff have a responsibility for their clinical practice, which requires them to ensure that every clinical interaction is evidence- and values-based. Healthcare is a very fluid environment that experiences continuous change, and therefore relying on what has been delivered historically will not always result in the provision of best care for the patient and service user.

Encouraging all staff to examine the research literature and discuss this with the patient will result in a service that is evidence- and values-based.

We furthermore suggest that healthcare professionals be mindful of the work of Bate and Robert (2007), who propose that service users ought to be engaged both at the micro level (co-designing their healthcare) and at the macro level (co-designing the service).

Staff should also be appraised of other aspects of clinical governance, such as risk management (for example, reporting near misses, raising and escalating concerns – including whistleblowing/speaking up), complaints management, and evaluation of practice through clinical audit and re-audit. However, these processes are often initiated and managed by more senior staff, including clinical governance leads.

Nonetheless, despite how committed and motivated healthcare staff are to continuously improve the quality of healthcare provision, there are numerous daily challenges that at times can be overwhelming. Throughout 2020 and 2021, the world has been faced with the COVID-19 pandemic and this has led to the lives of all healthcare staff becoming more challenging. One of the many consequences of a pandemic is its impact on stress and wellbeing. COVID-19 infection in healthcare workers is a major threat to both the individual and the service, not to mention their relatives who may be elderly, immunocompromised, or have chronic medical conditions. Stressful working environments and long working hours leading to fatigue and exhaustion, together with isolated related psychological factors, are affecting healthcare workers worldwide. Research undertaken in 2009 to assess the psychological impact of the 2003 outbreak of severe acute respiratory syndrome (SARS) on hospital employees in Beijing, China, showed that approximately 10% of participants included in the study ($n = 549$) had experienced high levels of post-traumatic stress (Wu *et al.*, 2009). Bearing in mind that during the period of infection from SARS, there were 8,098 reported cases and 774 deaths (NHS, 2020), it is a given that the psychological impact of COVID-19 will be much higher.

During 2020–2021, retired medics were asked to return to work, non-essential clinical work was abruptly halted, and seven Nightingale hospitals were opened in the UK. At least one suicide in the medical profession has been reported in America (Gulati and Kelly, 2020) and burnout amongst healthcare professionals is rife. The international political debate about the response to COVID-19 and who was responsible, at a governmental level, will no doubt continue for years.

COVID-19 has highlighted the need to keep staff safe, healthy, and well. Urgent action is also needed to address the systemic inequalities experienced by some NHS staff, particularly BAME staff (NHS, 2020).

There is also a need for better workforce planning and transformation to improve staff retention, encourage flexible working, and provide opportunities for developing and upskilling staff. Ongoing training and education, according to updated WHO and Centers for Disease Control protocols, is essential and must continue.

To summarize, much has been done to ensure that clinical governance is at the heart of healthcare practice, however, we believe that a further, and deeper, change in organizational culture and thinking is required. Improving the quality of healthcare provision is the responsibility of all members of staff and not just those with a recognized clinical governance remit. A change of thinking is required whereby transparency, openness, and candour become the new mantra for healthcare organizations.

References

Bate, P. and Robert, G. (2007) *Bringing User Experience to Healthcare Improvement: The concepts, methods and practices of experience-based design*. Oxford: Radcliffe Publishing.

Gulati, G. and Kelly, B.D. (2020) Physician suicide and the COVID-19 pandemic, *Occupational Medicine*, 70 (7): 514. Available at: https://doi.org/10.1093/occmed/kqaa104.

NHS (2020) *We are the NHS: People Plan for 2020/2021 – action for all of us*. Available at: https://www.england.nhs.uk/ournhspeople/ (accessed: 7 March 2021).

Ockenden Report (2020) *Maternity Services at the Shrewsbury and Telford Hospital NHS Trust*. Available at: https://assets.publishing.service.gov.uk/government/uploads/system/uploads/attachment_data/file/943011/Independent_review_of_maternity_services_at_Shrewsbury_and_Telford_Hospital_NHS_Trust.pdf (accessed: 7 March 2021).

Wu, P., Fang, Y., Guan, Z., Fan, B., Kong, J., Yao, Z. *et al.* (2009) The psychological impact of the SARS epidemic on hospital employees in China: Exposure, risk perception, and altruistic acceptance of risk, *Canadian Journal of Psychiatry*, 54 (5): 302–311.

Appendix

Suggested answers to questions posed in the chapters

Chapter 1

How does an understanding of the definitions of clinical governance help you develop your practice?	The definitions help you to understand that the clinical governance framework impacts on you, your patients, and your practice The definitions remind us that clinical governance is multifactorial and is everyone's responsibility, not just your manager's We therefore need to be engaged in audit, education and training, and CQI
Knowing that clinical governance is everyone's responsibility, how could you become more proactive in implementing your organization's strategy for quality improvement?	You could begin by accessing your organization's strategy and discussing with your line manager in your PDR. You could also discuss in team meetings
What is the role of the clinical governance lead in your organization?	
How do you feed into this role?	

Chapter 2

Does your place of work have clear policies pertaining to all of these issues? Do you know where to find them? Are they written in a language that is useful and meaningful to you?	These may be available as a hard copy or online, so do ensure you know how to access them If you do not find the language accessible, discuss in your team meetings or with your line manager how this could be resolved
Which aspects of the clinical governance framework could best be applied to assist with a reduction of incidence?	Using Som's definition of clinical governance, think about input, structure, processes, and outcomes CQI, education and training, risk management, evidence-based practice, and audit are key aspects of the clinical governance framework

Chapter 3

How do quality circles differ from focus groups?	Quality circles come together to discuss particular quality issues and begin to consider potential solutions. Focus groups do not deliver solutions; they are a means of eliciting views on a particular topic. Quality circles will result in an action plan; focus groups will not
Which would be your preferred tool?	This might depend on whether you have a preference for a visual representation of an issue or some other format

Chapter 4

What are the main barriers to change?	Resistance to change, disempowerment, uncertainty, and loss
Why does change need to be collaborative?	It is no longer appropriate for healthcare providers to adopt a paternalistic approach to care. Patients who are experts by experience need to be involved in the change process in order to become co-designers of their care
How do developmental, transitional, and transformational change differ?	*Developmental*: to improve current practice *Transitional*: the implementation of something different *Transformational*: the emergence of a new state, unknown until it takes shape
What are the key benefits and challenges when developing quality improvement programmes?	*Benefits*: improving the quality of patient care is one of the key benefits. Staff can also develop their own leadership, communication, project management, team working, and presentation skills *Challenges*: staff may not feel they can sustain changes to practice alongside other workplace pressures. If management are not supportive, then this will likely impact on the success of the programme

Chapter 5

What are the key differences between Schein's (2010) levels of culture?	The outside layer (artefacts) is visible unlike values, beliefs, and underlying assumptions. Decisions to join an organization might be made on a superficial basis (i.e. artefacts). Values, beliefs, and underlying assumptions can be understood only once employed in the organization

Which is the most inclusive of Handy's (1999) four cultural types?	Person culture
What is the disadvantage of this cultural type?	This may not be the best culture for a health or social care organization, because it lacks structure. The organization is subservient to the individual

Chapter 6

Why are EBP and VBP essential to clinical practice?	It is essential that all healthcare professionals understand current evidence in order to (a) challenge current outdated practice and (b) ensure that their practice is up to date The values of patients/service users and carers must be at the heart of everything we do
What is the difference between an integrated care pathway and a care bundle?	An integrated pathway identifies the steps of a patient's journey and which professional will carry out the task and provide timeframes Care bundles are a collection of interventions (usually three to five) that may be applied to the management of a particular condition
When examining your practice, what tool can help you ask an answerable question to ensure your practice is evidence-based?	PICOT
What do the letters PICOT stand for?	Depending on usage it could be: **P:** Patient or Population **I:** Intervention or Indicator **C:** Comparison or Control **O:** Outcome **T:** Time OR: **P:** Patient or Population **I:** Issue **C:** Context **O:** Outcome **T:** Time

Chapter 7

What is the key difference between quality assurance and CQI?	Quality assurance is a system whereby all procedures that have been designed and planned are followed. The quality assurance function should continually survey the quality philosophy of the organization. The quality assurance team is responsible for auditing all areas to highlight and correct errors CQI is the planning and execution of a flow of improvement to provide quality care that meets or exceeds expectation
What is the difference between quality assurance and risk management?	Quality assurance is about focusing on the delivery of quality care based on standards and measurable criteria Quality assurance focuses on problem identification, problem assessment, corrective action, follow-up, and reporting findings Risk management is the protection of assets and this is managed by risk identification, risk analysis, risk control or treatment, and risk financing
How does a poor complaints system impact on patients, carers, and staff?	Distress may be caused if the complaint is not dealt with swiftly, thoroughly, and transparently Dissatisfaction might occur if patients, carers, and staff do not know where to access the complaints policy or if it is not written in plain language Inadequate responses may cause distress and may exacerbate bereavement (Francis Report (2013) *Report of the Mid Staffordshire NHS Trust Foundation Trust Public Inquiry*. London: HMSO)

Chapter 8

What approach would you use when there has been an unexpected outcome to treatment given?	A critical incident audit
When might you undertake a retrospective audit?	Often using patient notes, when looking at what has happened in a particular area, for example the number of patient falls in the past six months

What are the advantages of audit?	Improve patient care Improve communication across clinical groups Increase professional satisfaction Improve administration
Name three barriers to clinical audit	Lack of resources; lack of expertise/advice in design and analysis; difficulties between groups and group members; lack of an overall plan for audit and organizational hindrance

Index

Printed and bound by CPI Group (UK) Ltd, Croydon, CR0 4YY

23/10/2025

01983038-0002